Sleep Comfy Now: Fix Sleep Disorders, Insomnia, and Find Rest

Table of Contents

Chapter 1: What Sleep is about

Sleep is a state of the body that everyone gets into for a number of hours every day, usually at night. When a person is in that state, the nervous system is dormant, eyes are closed, and the postural muscles are relaxed.

Also, the person's consciousness during that period is effectively suspended.

That condition – sleep – is crucial to the everyday routine of a person. In fact, on average, a person spends a third of the day asleep, and it is important that the sleep one enjoys is of good quality. This means getting sufficient sleep at the appropriate time.

Sleep is a necessity just like food, water, and other basic requirements of life. If you continually fail to get sufficient sleep, the brain is adversely affected in a way that the pathways that facilitate creation of fresh memories are interfered with.

Hence it becomes difficult for you to concentrate. Your response time to external stimuli also becomes delayed.

Sleep-related Physiology

Sleep helps to enhance different functions of the brain. This includes how neurons communicate amongst themselves.

A neuron is the brain's tiniest functional unit, a cell that is specially designed to communicate information to different cells of the nervous system and even to those of the glands and muscles.

In fact, although you are in a semi-conscious state when asleep, your body remains active alongside your brain, during which time any toxins that build up in your brain during the day are cleared.

While not everything about sleep's biological function is known, it is evident it has an effect on the systems of the body; the brain, heart, lungs, immune system, body metabolism, and others.

Research has shown that people who perennially get sleep of poor-quality face a greater risk of developing health disorders such as elevated blood pressure, diabetes, ailments of a cardiovascular nature, depression, and even obesity.

According to one expert at the University of Toronto, John Peever, and another one from Sunnybrook Health Sciences Center, Brian J.Murray, sleep plays an important role in helping the body to re-energize its cells and eliminate waste from within the brain.

These experts also reckon that sleep enhances a person's memory and capacity to learn, in addition to regulating the person's appetite, mood, and even libido.

Scientists have established that there are two types of sleep, one of them referred to as **SWS**, and the other **REM**.

The former, which is *Slow Wave Sleep*, is also termed *"deep sleep"*. The latter stands for *Rapid Eye Movement* and is also referred to as *"dreaming sleep"*.

Most of the time the moment people fall asleep they experience the SWS kind of sleep, which means at that time their brain is operating in big, slow waves as the body relaxes.

In the meantime, their breathing becomes deep, and that helps the brain and also the body to rebuild its strength following a long day of activity.

This recuperating process is crucial in enabling the person to be in shape to handle the following day's activities. The process of sleep is very complex and also dynamic, and it affects the way you feel and function.

In this chapter you will discover how sleep is naturally regulated, and what transpires within the brain as you sleep.

Sleep Anatomy

Among the brain structures involved in the process of sleep are the hypothalamus, brain stem, thalamus, pineal gland, basal forebrain, and the amygdale.

The hypothalamus
The hypothalamus is found deep within the brain, and its size is that of a peanut. It hosts nerve cells that are set in groups, which function as sleep control centers.

There are also some cell clusters known as SCN or Suprachiasmatic nucleus inside the hypothalamus, each of them with cells in the thousands. They act as information receptors that detect the light the eyes are exposed to.

The SCN is responsible for the control of the circadian rhythms, which is the sleeping-waking routine that corresponds to the night and day times.

There are cases where people have damaged SCN, and as a result their sleeping patterns become erratic. The reason for such sleeping inconsistencies is that such people's circadian rhythms are not in tandem with the cycle of light and darkness.

Many people who are visually impaired are still able to sense light, and hence they have capacity to modify their cycles of sleeping and waking up.

Brain Stem

A person's brain stem is at the bottom of the brain, and its role is to maintain communication with the hypothalamus to ensure the waking-sleeping transitions are under control.

This part of the brain is inclusive of some structures known as pons, midbrain, and medulla.

The cells inside the brain's hypothalamus and brain stem are responsible for promotion of sleep. They release some brain chemical known as GABA, which ends up reducing a person's arousal activity within these brain structures.

A person's brain stem, and particularly the medulla and pons, plays a particularly important role in the REM or Rapid Eye Movement sleep.

It signals the muscles responsible for proper posture of the body and movement of limbs to relax, so that one does not end up physically acting out his/her dreams.

The Thalamus

The thalamus is responsible for relaying information originating from the body senses right to the brain's cerebral cortex.

The cerebral cortex is that coating the brain has that is charged with interpreting and processing of information, so that it is converted from short-term to long-term memory.

Over sleep's several stages, the brain's thalamus remains quiet, so that you are able to shut out the external occurrences or the activities going on around you.

Nevertheless, the thalamus gets active in the REM sleep, as it sends out images and sounds as well as different sensations that end up filling one's dreams.

Pineal Gland

There is a part of the pineal gland in either of the two hemispheres of the brain.

This gland is a receptor of signals sent from the SCN or Suprachiasmatic nucleus, and its activity raises the production level of melatonin.

Melatonin is a hormone that enables one to sleep after lights have been turned off.

People whose sight is gravely impaired and are therefore unable to have a proper wake-sleep routine the natural way can improve their situation if they take small doses of melatonin at a fixed time every day, such as supplements containing this naturally occurring ingredient.

Basal Forebrain

This structure is found close to the front of the brain and also close to its bottom region. It is responsible for promotion of sleep as well as wakefulness.

Meanwhile, a section of a person's midbrain serves as his/her arousal system.

A person's sleep drive is supported by the discharge of a chemical known as adenosine, which is a by-product of the process of cellular energy consumption.

The chemical is released from various cells mainly within the basal forebrain.

The reason caffeine is known to counteract sleepiness is that it blocks the activity of the adenosine.

Amygdala

The brain's structure known as amygdala has an almond shape, and its role is to process emotions. This structure is most active when one is in the stage of REM sleep.

Important Mechanisms of Sleep

The major internal mechanisms of sleep that are biological in nature are two, one them the circadian rhythm and the other the homeostasis.

These work in tandem with each other for the sake of regulating the time you fall asleep and the moment you awake.

The Circadian Rhythm

The circadian rhythm directs a range of daily functions, which include fluctuations of wakefulness, temperature of your body, your metabolism, and even how the body releases various hormones.

It is this rhythm that controls when you feel sleepy and when you wake up and regulates this routine so that it ends up matching the night and day routines.

When your circadian rhythm is working optimally, you do not need an alarm clock to wake you up at daybreak.

It is important to note that the body has its own internal biological clock, and it is generally based on the normal day's 24 hour clock. This clock is responsible for controlling a person's circadian rhythm.

Although the circadian rhythm is synchronized with light and temperature as well as other factors within the environment, it is still operational even when none of those cues are present.

The Homeostasis

The homeostasis that is related to the routine of sleep and wakefulness is responsible for keeping track of a person's need to sleep.

Sleep drive of the homeostatic nature serves to remind the body that it should be asleep after the lapse of a particular length of time. It also regulates the intensity of sleep once the person has fallen asleep.

Homeostatic sleep drive becomes stronger as a person's hours of wakefulness pass, and it is this sleep "build-up" that is responsible for making you finally sleep deeply and for long.

Normally the more sleep deprived you are the more you are likely to sleep longer and heavily.

Nevertheless, other factors might influence how well the expected sleep-wakefulness routine works. These include any medications the individual is taking, the overall health of the person, the environment within which the person is trying to sleep, one's levels of stress, and even the kinds of food and drink one has consumed in a particular day before they sleep.

Among the most impactful factors is the presence of light.

The retina of the eye has cells that specialize in light detection, and they communicate to the brain if night has set in or daytime has arrived. These cells are, therefore, capable of delaying or advancing your wakefulness. Being exposed to light can interfere with how fast you fall asleep or how soon you awaken.

In daily life, people who work night shifts find it difficult to fall asleep once they proceed to bed, just as they find it a challenge to remain awake while at their workplace. This is because they are disrupting the natural sleep-wakefulness routine that is the circadian rhythm.

When people experience jet lag, it is because their circadian rhythms have been put out of sync with their usual "time zones" because time zones keep changing as people fly from country to country. Hence the passenger's internal clock is disrupted.

If a person's sleep-wakefulness routine is poorly aligned with his/her required durations of sleep, which means the person's internal clock and the real one are out of sync, the person can be said to have a disorder of the circadian rhythm.

In order to establish if one has a circadian rhythm disorder, there is a diagnostic system experts make use of known as the ICSD or *International Classification of Sleep Disorders* to help identify if an individual may be suffering from some sort of sleep disorder.

Chapter 2: Insomnia

The word 'insomnia' is derived from Latin where it means 'no sleep'. The term is used to define a person's inability to either fall asleep or even to maintain sleep.

Still, sometimes the term is used to refer to one's inability to refresh the body and mind even after being asleep for a good number of hours.

One neurology professor, Dr. Mark Mahowald, describes insomnia as the inability of a person to sustain sufficient sleep to make him/her feel well rested. Of all the sleep-related problems Americans complain about, insomnia rates the highest.

As per the national Center for Sleep Disorders Research that is within the NIH or National Institutes of Health, adults who complain of insomnia symptoms are between 30% and 40% on average every year.

Acute Insomnia

Sometimes the sleeping problem is acute, in which case it lasts a single night or several of them.

Incidences that lead to acute insomnia are often abrupt. Good examples are news that you are going to be *laid-off* from your job, loss of someone you care about, being caught up in a natural disaster, car accident, and such abrupt events that cause you extreme stress.

When you experience such stressful events, you could find it hard to fall asleep, and when you do it might become difficult to remain asleep for a reasonable period of time. This eventually leads to a poor quality of sleep, and consequently you are likely to be tired the following day.

According to the NIH, poor quality sleep can make you feel groggy when awake, and you may even find it difficult to concentrate.

There are also instances where acute insomnia causes anxiety and eventually leads to depression. The reverse also happens at times; anxiety leading to acute insomnia.

Chronic Insomnia

Other times people suffer from chronic insomnia, which means the sleep problem has lasted one or several months or even years.

In the US, those whose insomnia can be categorized as chronic are between 10% and 15%, and it is rare to find people who hardly have anything to complain about when it comes to their sleep patterns.

While a myriad of things can lead to chronic insomnia, often the culprit is some underlying medical problem.

Closely related are the medications that the person may be using, although stimulants have also been identified as common causes.

Still, some people suffer from chronic insomnia owing to the kind of lifestyle they lead.

Medical-related Causes

Several medical problems that cause insomnia are long-term in nature. They include respiratory problems like asthma, COPD or chronic obstructive pulmonary disease and sleep apnea.

Others are under cardiac ailments, such as congestive heart failure.

Other long-term medical ailments that often lead to chronic insomnia include diabetes, fibromyalgia, and acid reflux, as well as restless leg syndrome, hyperthyroidism and urinary incontinence.

Chronic pain can also cause chronic insomnia, and so can conditions of anxiety, bipolar disorder, physical or emotional stress, and even depression.

Menopause is another culprit when it comes to causing chronic insomnia, and so are the diseases of Alzheimer's and Parkinson's.

Insomnia Causing Medications

Among the categories of medications likely to cause chronic insomnia are anti-depressants and beta-blockers; diuretics; drugs for chemotherapy; and medications that contain pseudoephedrine used to treat colds and allergies.

Insomnia Causing Stimulants

The stimulants likely to cause chronic insomnia include alcohol, nicotine and caffeine; illicit drugs like cocaine; and also, stimulants used as laxatives.

Insomnia Causing Lifestyle Patterns

Some of the common patterns of lifestyle likely to lead to chronic insomnia are working in shifts of a rotating nature; traveling frequently across varying time zones, a habit that leads to hours of jetlag; being physically inactive; taking frequent naps during the day; sleeping in an environment not conducive for sleep; and not having a sleep-wake routine.

Intermittent Insomnia

What seems to be prevalent in the US is a situation where people have serious problems sleeping for a couple of nights and then following that with a series of nights where their sleep is sufficient.

In short, the lack of proper sleep in this case is on and off. This kind of problem is referred to as chronic-intermittent insomnia.

The period intermittent insomnia lasts is usually below one week and sometimes two on the higher side, and the condition does not normally need medical intervention.

If, for instance, the reason for this intermittent insomnia is jetlag that ends up disrupting your sleep-wake cycle, your biological clock soon gets back to its normal functioning sleep wake cycles after a certain period of time.

However, there are cases where individuals experience sleepiness during the day and hence have poor work performance, and such people can benefit from use of *sleeping pills* as long as they use them on a short-term basis.

Such medications are meant only to enhance the person's sleep so that he/she can be alert enough to work the following day.

Nevertheless, it needs to be noted that there are risks involved with the use of *sleeping pills* bought over the counter, and as such medical practitioners generally discourage it.

Negative Impact of Insomnia

The problem of insomnia does not only disrupt your everyday life due to poor focus that can make you prone to accidents, it is also frustrating. Lying in bed for hours on end hoping to fall asleep can easily cause you anxiety.

Research conducted at the department of Health Services within the University of Wisconsin indicates that people who suffer from insomnia happen to be five times at risk of developing anxiety disorders and even depression.

The report also indicates that the risk such people have of suffering congestive heart failure as well as diabetes is twice as high.

Worse still, their risk of becoming dependent on alcohol and even drugs is seven times as high compared to people with healthy sleep patterns.

Erratic sleep patterns are not just bad for mental health, but they are also bad for physical as well as emotional health.

Also, insomnia's negative health effects have ripple effects on the individual's other spheres of life like education, career, and even their social life.

In fact, experts have found that insomnia has significant consequences on society in general.

In this chapter, you will see the effects insomnia has on a person's health, and what it does to his/her social and economic spheres of life.

Social Consequences of Insomnia

There are several social consequences of insomnia, and they include poor quality of one's life.

Since people with insomnia have an elevated risk of falling and getting hip fractures, their health as well as their social life is likely to deteriorate.

It is, for example, impossible for a person who is physically incapacitated to go out socializing, and this therefore affects the person's social life.

Also, when a person is groggy from lack of sleep, he/she is unlikely to be either a good guest or a dependable host.

Besides, people with sleep deficiencies are known to be easily irritable and hence poor company.

Economic Consequences of Insomnia

Insomnia is not only a social problem but also an economic one. The fact that with insomnia one can barely focus on the job at hand means that his/her productivity is bound to be adversely affected.

If the proportion of employees with chronic or even intermittent insomnia is big, the business for which they work is likely to incur cumulative losses not only in terms of lost hours, but also in reduced efficiencies.

Tangible output might drop, and for goods being produced the level of rejects and inaccuracies might end up increasing.

The relationship between hours slept and work performance has become somewhat complicated over the years.

As the industrial revolution set in, capitalism including machines, infrastructure and electricity expanded all over the country, and was embraced for enabling a 24-hour economy, it also meant that companies and individuals were tempted to work longer periods to increase productivity.

This reality has helped individuals to increase their incomes and helped the economy to grow, but in turn it has also meant employees, managers and CEOs are sleeping fewer hours in most cases.

Data derived from the US Bureau of Labor Statistics in 2016 indicated that more people now go home with work to do, as opposed to switching off from work mode when they leave the office or work environment.

It was also reported that on average, an American does four and a half hours of work from home every week, in addition to his/her official working hours.

However, 20% of Americans spend ten hours at the minimum every week working from home in addition to their official working hours.

Other researchers whose focus was on managers found that in the UK the work the managers do after office hours is equivalent to the length of their respective annual leaves.

This then means that when ultimately the individual takes his/her annual leave, the break does not serve the purpose it was originally meant to serve, but rather just saves the individual from burnout and fatigue.

Excessive Work at the Expense of Sleep

A research study conducted in twelve countries to find out how working longer affects sleep established that for every extra hour an employee works, it reduces his/her capacity to sleep by ten minutes.

Researchers were also quick to point out that such reduction of sleep has a negative impact on productivity.

The end result, therefore, is that increment in revenues earned by the company does not correspond to the extra hours the employees put in.

A survey done at Harvard University involving 7,400 subjects found that deprivation of sleep ends up costing companies around $2,280 for every one of its employees, or $11^{1}/_{3}$ days of productivity annually.

From that study, it was estimated that the country loses as much as $63.2 billion every year just from shortcomings associated with sleep deprivation.

Researchers who based their study on Australia estimated that the country's annual losses from insomnia are close to one percent of the economy's GDP or Gross Domestic Product. In short, insomnia is a global challenge.

A review done by RAND on five of the thirty-five countries that comprise the Organization for Economic Co-operation and Development or OECD established that losses in productivity that emanate from insomnia-related challenges run into hundreds of billions when the estimates are made in dollars.

RAND, whose full name is Research and Development, is a non-profit organization whose aim is to enhance policy as well as decision making by way of research and proper analysis.

From the research findings, it is understandable why countries like the US and Japan that are among the most greatly affected by insomnia have the greatest number of citizens suffering from sleep deprivation.

It has been established that the number of hours half of the adults in these countries enjoy are below the hours health experts have recommended, which are between *7 and 8* per 24-hour day.

When people are deprived of sleep, their immune system is easily compromised, and they are therefore likely to fall ill faster compared to someone who gets adequate sleep.

In fact, people who are perennially deprived of sleep are three times more likely to catch the common cold than those who consistently have adequate sleep.

As would be expected, the more people become ill the more they take time off work and the more overall business productivity drops.

As for the individuals, their career lives end up becoming shorter, which not only adversely affects the individual but the economy as well.

Diagnosis of Insomnia

There are different ways of diagnosing insomnia, and the physician may decide to use more than one approach in order to understand your situation as an individual.

At the end the remedy your physician recommends may be one you can implement at home, one that requires a clinic appointment, or a combination of both remedies.

In many cases the physician will ask you questions pertaining to your experience with regards to sleep, your daily routine, significant events that may have taken place in your life, and such others.

Depending on the answers you provide or the observations he/she makes during the assessment, the physician might recommend some blood tests, and other times he/she might propose admission to the hospital so that your sleep pattern can be studied overnight.

If deemed appropriate physicians may prescribe pharmaceutical grade medications or drugs to help alleviate insomnia symptoms short term.

The reason the physician would wish to do a proper evaluation and assessment of you is so as to understand what your unique experience entails, which would then make it possible to prescribe the most suitable plan of treatment.

Major Approaches to Insomnia Diagnosis

Maintenance of a Sleep Log

Sleep logs refers to a basic diary where you keep track of every detail pertaining to your sleeping habits.

In your logs you record the time you go to bed, the time you wake up, the intensity of sleepiness you experience at varying times of the day, and any other significant things pertaining to your experience with sleep.

Normally the physician prefers that you maintain the sleep log for around two weeks, with the shortest period being one week.

This record helps the physician to understand your sleep problem with relative clarity.

It is recommended that you fill in your sleep log as soon as you wake up so that you record your nighttime and morning experiences when they are still fresh in your mind.

The information sought in the sleep log includes when you put out the lights at night, the kind of beverages you had taken especially if they are caffeinated, when you last had a meal and what size it was, what your experience is of the quality of sleep you had, and so on.

You can make use of phone apps, such as notepads or journals that serves the same purpose as the manual sleep log, if you find that more convenient.

Completion of a Sleep Inventory

Sleep inventory refers to an elaborate questionnaire designed to assemble information regarding your health, your medical history, and even your sleep patterns.

Among the questions in the questionnaire is your basic complaint regarding sleep, your family status in terms of spouse and children, how often you awake at night and how long it takes you to feel sleepy again, whether you snore, snort or gasp as you sleep, whether you suffer headaches in the morning, and such other questions.

Use of Blood Tests

Sometimes physicians find it necessary to carry out blood tests to find out if there are any medical issues underlying the sleeping disorder.

For example, problems of the thyroid are often disruptive to sleep, and if it is discovered you have such a problem, the doctor can treat it first before addressing the problem of sleep.

Other laboratory tests the physician might order include an assessment of iron levels, signs of stimulants or opiates in the body, or even significant levels of anti-anxiety medications.

The reason doctors are interested in learning if the patient has been using these medications mentioned is because they are notorious for affecting a person's alertness level, and as a consequence the ability to sleep normally.

Other Sleep Disorder Diagnostic Tests
Overnight Oximetry

Among the easiest diagnostic tests to carry out is the overnight oximetry. It is also one of the tests many physicians like to carry out in their assessment of the patient's sleeping problem.

Overnight oximetry is a procedure where the patient wears a probe either on his/her finger, or even on the earlobe, for the purpose of gauging how well the blood is oxygenated.

This probe also has capacity to assess the patient's heart rate.

Also, the gadget has a red light as well as a sensor, which serve to detect any color changes that occur in the blood. Some color changes may denote de-saturation, meaning the level of oxygen in the blood is falling.

This test helps to indicate if you are at risk of experiencing nighttime breathing problems such as sleep apnea.

It also helps the physician determine whether you require extra evaluation like polysomnogram, a test abbreviated as PSG.

The PSG

PSG is widely considered the gold standard when it comes to diagnosing a sleep disorder.

Evaluation entails a sleep-over at one of the sleep centers available, where a technician specially trained in the area of sleep disorders monitors you.

In some cases, the sleep center, sometimes referred to as a sleep laboratory, is within a hospital.

Among the data recorded during the overnight monitoring in a sleep center are physiological parameters of EEG and EKG, respiration, level of oxygen, muscle tone, as well as movement of the eyes and of other extremities.

Your entire night's sleep is also recorded on audio and video for the physician to analyze later.

The data recorded during this overnight stay helps to diagnose a range of sleep disorders such as sleep apnea, parasomnias, restless legs syndrome, and others.

The Titration Study

This study is usually referred to as the CPAP titration study, and it is often performed alongside the PSG.

The reason these tests are done together is to utilize time efficiently and minimize the medical bill, save the patient from the suspense of waiting for different results in sequence, and enable the physician to initiate treatment as soon as possible.

CPAP stands for Continuous Positive Airway Pressure (CPAP), a form of therapy used in the treatment of obstructive sleep apnea. When conditions like sleep apnea are treated early, the risk of the patient developing cardiovascular illnesses is minimized.

In this titration study, the technician increases CPAP pressure via a soft mask on a gradual basis, a process that ends up eliminating most episodes where breathing could cease.

When the optimal level is identified, it is recorded so that it can be recommended to the patient during home therapy.

For smooth running of the titration test, the technician often observes the patient's pattern of breathing from an adjacent room. The reason the technician works from a distance is to avoid disturbing the patient as he or she works.

They then continue to make adjustments to the settings in an upward direction as need be as the patient sleeps. The technician sets the CPAP pressure low at the beginning of the night, or what is termed as bi-level.

Then as the patient falls asleep the technician monitors him/her so as to identify incidences of breathing disruptions.

In case hypopneas or apneic incidences are observed, or even snoring, the technician remotely adjusts the CPAP machine pressure upwards.

Monitoring continues thereafter with the goal of elimination of snoring and minimization of incidences of apnea or even hypopnea.

While a person fails to breath in conditions of sleep apnea, the airway is only partially blocked in cases of hypopnea.

From the distant location of the technician, he/she observes the patient and notes how long the deep sleep lasts, and the duration of the rapid eye movement.

It is recommended that the patient be in the supine position as the test is carried out. This is the position where one lies on the back, and it is in this position that sleep apnea is at its worst.

Multiple Sleep Latency Testing

Multiple Sleep Latency Testing that is abbreviated as MSLT is often referred to as 'nap study'. The way it is set up is similar to the setup of PSG, a test already described in the chapter.

MSLT is normally carried out after the patient has already undergone the PSG study conducted overnight.

It is after the patient has woken up from the night of sleep monitoring that he/she is scheduled for a day of nap times, during which he/she is monitored in spans of two hours each.

Ordinarily, a patient undergoing this testing is directed to bed and let to lie in it for twenty minutes, with the hope that before that time lapses, he/she will have fallen asleep.

All the while there is a technician monitoring the patient so as to identify the patient's sleep onset, and to particularly note the period of REM sleep.

The patient is woken up when the 20-minute period lapses, but after a period of two hours he/she is directed to bed again. This process of 20-minute naps after every two hours is repeated for a period covering more than ten hours.

The essence of this testing is to identify the patient's excessive sleepiness during the day, which presents in a variety of ways. Some patients manifest sleep apnea; others idiopathic hypersomnia, which means sleeping excessively within good reason; while still others manifest narcolepsy.

The condition of narcolepsy is not only marked by extreme sleepiness, but it is also indicated by paralysis and even hallucinations.

At times the patient even experiences episodes where control of muscles is partially or fully lost; a condition known as cataplexy. Strong emotions like laughter or anger are known for being common triggers of cataplexy.

The MWT Approach

This approach of MWT or Maintenance of Wakefulness assesses the person's capacity to remain awake for a specified duration of time.

During this test, the patient is given a place to lie but asked to remain awake. The technician observes the person for forty minutes, and if that person does not have excessive or extreme sleepiness, he/she is able to remain awake for the timed forty-minute period.

In comparison, while MWT tests a person's capacity to remain awake or alert during the day, MSLT tests a person's level of sleepiness during a similar period.

Actigraphy

In actigraphy, the patient with sleeping issues has activity measurements taken using a tiny device the size of a wristwatch. The device is wrapped around the person's wrist so that it can pick up signals that indicate the presence of movement.

If no signals are detected, or just a few of them are picked up, it means the person is fast asleep or at full rest.

This means the devise has the capacity to provide information on the times when the person has slept well or has been well rested. The duration patients are required to wear the device varies in length depending on what the physician thinks an individual patient requires according to their assessments.

The activities measured through actigraphy are actually movements that indicate the patient's sleep-waking cycles or what is termed the circadian rhythm. This is observed over a long time, which may extend to weeks or in some cases, months.

The tiny device used helps in determining if the patient is experiencing any disruptions in his/her sleep-wake cycles. The reason physicians are interested in finding out if the patient is affected by such disruptions is that they are very prevalent in people who have sleep disorders associated with their circadian rhythm.

Examples of circadian rhythm disorders include ASPD and DSPS, which stand for Advanced Sleep Phase Disorder and Delayed Sleep-Phase Syndrome respectively. Sometimes ASPD is referred to as ASPT, which stands for Advanced Sleep-Phase Type.

A person affected by DSPS experiences sleep delays of two hours or more beyond normal sleeping time.

Insomnia is another example of a circadian rhythm disorder. The rate of activity measured in actigraphy is usually correlated with the patient's sleep diary.

Chapter 3: Stress, Trauma & PSTD in relation to Insomnia

Sleep disorders are prevalent in the US. According to the CDC or the Center for Disease Control, around a third of all Americans in the adult demographic have complained of not having sufficient sleep, a situation that the organization has termed an *epidemic*.

Sleep onset insomnia, meaning inability to sleep when needed, and sleep maintenance insomnia, meaning inability to remain asleep at nighttime, are the two major conditions responsible for the sleep disorder epidemic people are facing.

It has also been noted that many Americans consider themselves as having high stress levels, something that the APA or American Psychiatric Association has ascertained in some of their annual surveys.

It is therefore understandable that many adults would find it difficult to enjoy quality sleep.

Worry, anger, anxiety, and other emotions associated with stress have a direct link to unhealthy sleep patterns or the sheer inability to sleep.

Studies conducted by the CDC have shown that 35.2% of US adults sleep below 7 hours every night, which can easily lead to accumulated sleep deficit likely to develop into a full blown physical or even mental ailment.

Although it is often difficult to spell out the specific role that sleep plays in overall health, it is clear that some mental and physiological processes work more efficiently when one has been sleeping adequately.

Such processes that keep you physically and mentally fit include muscle repair and mental relaxation. They are great for relaxing your body and mind.

Negative   Impact   of Inadequate Sleep

People who are deprived of sleep are at a high risk of depression, among other ailments. The conditions begin with being consistently in a foul mood, feeling lethargic, being unable to concentrate, making poor judgments, and being generally incapable of operating normally.

At the workplace, if you have been sleep deprived, you can end up making poor decisions in matters that are so crucial that you cause the your employer or business huge monetary losses.

Incidentally, people in positions of power have been found to be the most adversely affected by sleep related problems. Research has found that half of the CEOs in the top fortune 500 companies sleep less than six hours every night.

Further research indicates that the higher up the corporate ladder you are the higher are your earnings, but the fewer hours you can sleep.

It is apparent that while stress levels are often a cause of insomnia, the converse is also true. The professionals who have a bigger stake to lose if the company performs poorly often get stressed more than the average worker, and therefore their sleep is disrupted at night.

At the same time, because of the long hours these high-performance individuals work, they cannot afford to sleep long hours. After all, their minds are always set on the moves they are going to make the following day to propel the company forward.

Consistent lack of sufficient sleep then leads to fatigue and a build-up of physical and mental stress.

Studies have shown that CEOs and chairpersons of big corporations sleep a mere six and a quarter of an hour each day, while senior managers sleep just three minutes longer.

In the meantime, first line managers in the same company sleep for six hours and twenty-five minutes each day, the individual professional six hours and thirty-three minutes, while the average employee is able to enjoy a good seven hours and fifty minutes.

According to CEO Coaching International, top performing CEOs are on the path to dying silently from stress.

Nevertheless, this organization of professionals reckons that this unfortunate state of affairs does not have to be. Their advice to CEOs and others with demanding jobs is to let go of anything that can distract an hour before sleep time. This includes games, TV and even movies.

Effect of Trauma on Sleep

One of the adverse effects of trauma is problems falling asleep or problems sleeping long and well enough. Trauma in this case does not refer to physical injury, but to an extremely distressing experience.

Such greatly disturbing experiences are generally grouped into three categories, one of them being acute trauma. Acute trauma is a result of a one-off distressing incident.

For example, if one is involved in a serious car accident where one or more people lost their lives, the horror of what the person witnessed might remain with him/her for a long time.

Another category is the chronic trauma, where distressing incidences keep recurring in a person's life, or probably at one time in life they kept recurring. These can be well exemplified by domestic abuse of different kinds, including physical violence.

The third category is the complex trauma, where one has undergone a range of traumatic experiences that involve other people and for a prolonged time, with minimal or no hope of getting out of the situation.

People ordinarily develop complex trauma after undergoing experiences such as persistent family violence, sexual trafficking, or even genocide.

When one undergoes a traumatizing experience, the body becomes over-stimulated, with excessive neuro-chemicals flooding the brain; the kind that keeps one awake, like epinephrine, adrenaline, and such others. The effect of this overstimulation is that it is not easy from that point onwards to catch sleep.

These neuro-chemicals do not leave the brain, and so even when the body is exhausted and you decide to lie down, rest and eventually fall sleep, the normal sleep pattern keeps being interrupted by the abundance of the neuro-chemicals in the brain.

That is how one ends up suffering insomnia out of trauma, and for those who escape trauma they usually have unpleasant dreams. Ultimately, such a person is bound to experience fatigue during the day because the system never really rested.

Trauma-related Sleep Challenges

Among the problems people are likely to experience after undergoing trauma are flashbacks, meaning they visualize the disturbing experiences they went through or witnessed.

They could also be plagued with disturbing thoughts related to those bad experiences of the past. Sometimes victims of trauma feel like they need to be always alert, and this alertness makes it difficult for them to catch sleep.

For people who have particularly lived in violent environments, their level of anxiety often rises when night falls and it becomes dark; they become excessively restless and this interferes with their capacity to sleep.

When a person in such a situation manages to fall asleep, he/she is likely to experience nightmares, and since these are usually frightening, the person is jerked into consciousness and finds it very hard to resume sleep.

Unfortunately, many people who have trouble sleeping because of trauma try to find respite in alcohol, because drinking tends to numb them to sleep.

However, since alcohol induced sleep can only last a few hours, these trauma survivors end up not only with insufficient sleep but also sleep of poor quality. This is because the processes that take place in the brain when one is sober or not very drunk may be interfered with when senses are numbed by alcohol.

Research studies show that while drinking alcohol may help healthy people fall to sleep faster and even sleep more heavily, it does reduce the individual's sleep phase of rapid eye movement, or REM. This is the phase where a person experiences dreams.

How well one sleeps during this phase that comes one and a half hours after falling asleep is of great significance, because this period is thought to contribute to the restoration of a person's brain health.

In fact, after sleep has been interrupted in the REM phase, people tend to be drowsy the following day and do not concentrate very well.

According to Irshaad Ebrahim, a medical researcher who has served as medical director at UK's London Sleep Center, alcohol disrupts sleep yet this may not be apparent because of its sleep inducing effect; and it also precipitates sleep apnea because of its tendency to suppress a person's breathing.

Nevertheless, Ebrahim points out that a standard drink or two do not affect sleep in any significant manner, otherwise the more people drink before going to bed, the more likely they are to experience sleep disruptions.

Ebrahim also warns that those who regularly rely on alcohol to fall asleep quickly risk becoming alcohol dependent, yet for a good part of the night their sleep will still be disrupted.

Ebrahim's sentiments have been echoed by Scott Krakower, an expert in addiction at New York's North Shore-LIJ, who says it is a misconception to think that alcohol enhances sleep. North Shore-LIJ is a health provider based in New York.

Dr. Michael Breus who is a sleep expert from Scottsdale, Arizona is another professional who holds a similar position on alcohol use.

He reckons that because REM is responsible for restoring a person's mental health, once it is continually interrupted through alcohol use, some other health risks become greater, including the tendency to sleepwalk or sleep talk.

He notes also that one is likely to develop memory problems if the sleep problems persist unchecked.

Due to the risks involved, experts discourage people from using alcohol to try and numb pain experienced out of trauma. Specifically, they say not only can alcohol interfere with the people's recovery process, but their sleep issues can also be exacerbated.

The Effect of PTSD on Insomnia

PTSD is an acronym for Post Traumatic Stress Disorder, a health condition of a psychological nature that sets in following a traumatizing event.

A person with PTSD keeps having unpleasant experiences, often disturbing, which elicit the kinds of emotions one experiences as a result of trauma. Such feelings include fear, horror, and a sense of helplessness, and they need to be addressed.

Some of the distressing events that cause PTSD include involvement in military combat or sudden loss of someone dear. Such events cause temporary anxiety at first, but then thoughts of the distressing incident keep recurring and they lead to insomnia.

PTSD usually develops in two stages, the first one having symptoms that last up to three months after the disturbing event. This form of PTSD is referred to as acute PTSD. The second stage is referred to as chronic PTSD, and here symptoms last for more than three months after the distressing event.

It is said that roughly seven to eight percent of people end up with PTSD at various stages of life, and prevalence is higher in women than in men when the underlying cause is domestic violence or assault of a sexual nature. PTSD sometimes exists alongside depression.

Categories of PTSD Symptoms

While the underlying cause of PTSD is the existence of distressing events, the disorder may manifest differently in different people. Hence, PTSD symptoms are divided into three categories.

One of them is termed 're-experience', another 'avoidance', and lastly 'hyper-arousal'.

Major Symptoms of Re-experiencing PTSD
People with the re-experiencing form of PTSD have symptoms like recollections of the grave events of the past, which include associated thoughts or perceptions and even images, dreams, and also nightmares.

They end up re-living the distressing experiences and having illusions and hallucinations associated with them, and sometimes they have flashbacks.

Major Symptoms of Avoidance PTSD

People with the avoidance PTSD do their best to avoid any reminders of those events that caused them trauma; anything likely to trigger those distressing memories.

Among the things they avoid are places and people who in one way or another reawaken the disturbing emotions. Often they also suppress thoughts and feelings similar to the ones they felt when the bad events took place.

They even avoid conversations and activities either linked to those traumatizing events, or that somehow become a reminder of that unfortunate past.

People affected in this way are often detached as they relate to others who have nothing to do with their past experiences, and sometimes they even get estranged from people otherwise close to them.

Major Symptoms of Hyper-arousal PTSD

Insomnia is a major symptom among people suffering hyper-arousal, but there are also other symptoms involved like irritability and inability to concentrate.

People with hyper-arousal PTSD are also prone to angry outbursts, and they are easily startled. They are also hyper-vigilant, behaving as if they do not trust the environment they are in.

When one is hyper-vigilant, his/her sensory sensitivity is elevated; and related behavior, such as an attempt to detect intrusion, is intensified.

This often makes the person so anxious that it causes him/her great exhaustion. Furthermore, hyper-arousal has a way of making someone paranoid.

Some people even unconsciously fight sleep for fear of being attacked when they are not self-aware, and they end up sleeping very lightly. This means they are conscious of every little noise that occurs within the house. If this state of affairs persists, the person's problem of insomnia becomes very difficult to solve.

Associated with this category of hyper-arousal PTSD is isolated sleep paralysis, abbreviated as ISP, which sets in as soon as sleep begins or as soon as one has awoken from sleep.

By sleep paralysis is meant the inability to move even when there is nothing wrong with the senses; so the person is no longer asleep and is somewhat aware of the surroundings, but feels like heavy pressure is being exerted to make him/her immobile. In some cases, the person feels like choking.

Clearly, the effects of PTSD are several and some are very serious, and those associated with sleep include insomnia, nightmares and ISP. Various surveys have shown that of all the people suffering PTSD, 70% of them have sleep-related complaints that include insomnia as well as nightmares.

PTSD-related nightmares involve fresh experiences involving past disturbing events, which can sometimes be very vivid and easy to recall when one awakens.

Some of these experiences involve the person moving around or doing some activity, in their sleep or as they transition to the state of wakefulness. Some people with this behavior also sleep talk.

What is most unfortunate about these PTSD-related symptoms is that they may lead to violent behavior or behavior that can easily cause injury to one-self or someone else.

Some people with PTSD try to fight the symptoms by indulging in alcohol, but just like in the case of trauma-related sleep problems, drinking alcohol is not helpful. Instead, one begins to experience sleep apnea or intermittent sleep disruptions.

Treating PTSD-related insomnia can be problematic, as even the observations made in sleep laboratories have not brought out any significant anomalies in the behavior of the subjects studied.

Generally what has been observed is an increase in movements during sleep and disordered or fragmented REM sleep, and even these findings are not consistent in all the individuals studied.

This means it is important that experts continue to study the symptoms of PTSD-related sleep disorders, so that it can become easier to seek effective solutions.

Chapter 4: How Dreams Affect Sleep

It is important to learn something about dreams because they occur when one is asleep, and the major topic of this book is sleep and related problems.

According to the US National Sleep Foundation, everyone gets to dream in their sleep whether they recall it or not, because this is a normal feature of sleep.

The foundation points out that in a single night, an average person dreams for a total of two hours, and this dreaming can take place at any of the normal stages of sleep. This means the healthy process of dreaming can be interfered with owing to sleep disruptions at any of the stages.

Nevertheless, the REM sleep phase is the one most affected, because it is during this phase that dreams are most vivid. How dreams happen in this phase affects how relaxed you feel when you arise or how disturbed you feel.

How Sleep Progresses to the REM Phase

The REM sleep is the phase of sleep that begins an hour and a half into falling sleep. A person experiences several changes of a physiological nature during this period.

These changes include relaxation of the muscles, movement of the eyes, increased pace of respiration, and elevated level of brain activity. The REM phase comes after a person has reached and passed the stage of deep NREM sleep, which is also referred to as 'stage 3' of sleep.

Importance of the NREM Sleep Phase
NREM is an acronym for Non-Rapid Eye Movement, and it is the period of sleep during which the most intense restoration takes place. Once a person has entered this sleep stage, it is very difficult to awaken him/her.

The NREM phase of sleep has its own three stages, one whose duration ranges from five to fifteen minutes. During this initial stage, a person's eyes are shut but it is still easy to tap him/her into consciousness.

In the second stage of NREM, the sleep is light with the rate of heartbeat much slower and the temperature of the body lower as well. These changes happen as the body prepares to enter the phase where sleep is quite deep – the third stage.

This third stage of NREM is where sleep is so deep that arousing someone is very hard; and if you succeed in doing so the person is visibly disoriented for a number of minutes.

It is during this stage when the body repairs itself and reproduces new tissue, constructs bones, and also works towards strengthening the entire immune system.

How Dreaming is affected in the REM Phase

The initial stage of the REM phase ordinarily lasts around ten minutes, but REM's subsequent stages becomes progressively longer as one continues to sleep; the last stage can even last one complete hour.

During this time, the person's rate of heartbeat continues to increase and the respiration rate increases as well.

It is the stage during which the brain is most active and dreams at this stage are often intense.

There is a part of a person's brain known as 'pons', and this is the place where sleep signals originate from during REM.

This part is responsible for shutting off the signals previously reaching the spinal cord, so they do not get there during REM.

The shutting off of these signals is what makes a person's body entirely immobile at the REM phase of sleep.

This means then that in case pons does not disconnect the signals going to the spinal cord, the person will end up acting out his/her dreams.

To make it easy to understand REM, Rubin Naiman who is a psychologist and a specialist in dreams provides a clear explanation. He says REM should be viewed as not happening in one continuous period, but in different stages of sleep throughout the night.

The stages that happen during the initial two-thirds of a person's sleep are individually relatively short, and this is because the body gives priority to sleep that is deep and slow in waves.

The more lengthy stages of REM occur in the last sleeping hours, which, for the majority of people, is early in the morning.

Professor Naiman, who is based at the University of Arizona's Center for Integrative Medicine, observes that for people who do not sleep the recommended time of seven to eight hours, they miss the chance to enjoy the last stage of REM.

On the overall, a person goes through cycles of NREM and REM in alternating order, with dreams occurring during the REM phase.

The REM sleep Behavior Disorder

Normally a person's senses are at rest when one is asleep, and considering they all work together when one is awake, it is very risky to have only the signals that trigger acting out working in isolation.

With no other senses to give the person some coordination, one ends up moving with no sense of direction and can ram into a wall or trip down a staircase.

This behavior is a rare sleep disorder known as The REM Sleep Behavior Disorder.

Effect of Sleep Disturbance in REM

It is important to note that the sections of a person's brain that are active during the REM phase of sleep are associated with enhancing capacity to learn and remember.

Experts see that fact as explaining the reason infants end up learning a lot even before they can speak, considering half of their sleep is spent in the REM phase.

For adults, only a fifth of their sleeping time is spent in the REM phase but it is still impactful. This has been proven in cases where a person is taught certain skills in the day but then is deprived of sleep during what would have been the REM phase.

Such an individual hardly remembers what had earlier been taught.

Overall Effect of Dreams on Health

Dreams are considered to be one of the ways a person's brain consolidates its memories. It is said that dreamtime is when a person's brain re-organizes and reviews the events of the day, and connects them to earlier experiences.

However, there are those experts who believe in what is termed the 'activation synthesis theory, who consider dreams to be attempts made by the brain to find some logic in signals that appear randomly as one sleeps.

Under this theory, the belief is that there are people who have capacity to control the direction their dreams take, and for them the subject matter of their dream is mostly influenced by the thoughts they had latest before falling asleep.

Whatever dreams one has, the wish would be they did not interrupt sleep, so that the person can wake up relaxed and refreshed.

Nevertheless, this is not sometimes the case especially when the dreams are scary. These tend to linger on one's mind to the following day, interfering with one's mood and mental state of health.

In the immediate time, one is unable to fall back to sleep after being interrupted by an unpleasant dream, and this causes what is sometimes referred to as 'bad-dream hangover'.

Luckily, dreams do not affect the architecture of sleep, so that for those whose dreams come before NREM or even REM, as long as one manages to fall back asleep, they are still able to enjoy the rich and relaxing phases.

Study findings appearing on the Journal of Neuroscience indicated that people who enjoyed a lot of their sleep in the REM phase where most dreaming takes place, manifest less of the brain activity associated with fear. This observation was made after these people had been subjected to moderate electric shocks after a night of nice sleep.

Experts therefore hypothesized that having a good night's sleep with uninterrupted REM a day prior to undergoing a scary experience, might save people from developing PTSD.

These are some of the reasons the sleeping environment should be conducive to falling asleep; being without streaks of light and interrupting noises.

In general, people who have pleasant dreams report feeling happy and well rested the following day, while people who have disturbing dreams report feeling uneasy and still tired the following day.

The converse is true; people who are happy report having had pleasant dreams and those who are unhappy and under stress report having had unpleasant dreams.

Experts have not yet established which one is the cause – one's state in the day or the dreams that occur in the night – hence seeing it as an 'egg and chicken' situation.

In the meantime, it would appear that working towards minimizing stress and preparing well for a good night's sleep would enhance the quality of sleep and contribute to a person's overall health.

The Connection between Sleep and Immunity

There is a strong link between the quality of sleep a person enjoys and the state of immunity of such a person.

Dr. Diwakar Balachandran of Houston's University of Texas, confirms this. Statistics by the Center for Disease Control or CDC has shown that adult Americans with sleep disorders are in the millions – ranging from fifty to seventy million.

This means the country's healthcare system could be relieved of a significant burden if only more people would manage to sleep a minimum of seven hours of quality sleep, which would then translate to higher productivity in the day and an improved economy.

Although it is not easy to spell out the direct link between sleep and immunity, the fact that the body and the mind are repaired during sleep is enough to affirm the existence of an important relationship.

Also, since the immune system contains the cells and the proteins responsible for fighting off colds and flu, it means if it becomes weak owing to lack of sufficient sleep the health of a person is bound to be compromised.

In fact, Dr. Balachandran asserts that a person's T-cells drop in number when he/she is deprived of sleep; and in the meantime the cytokines linked to inflammation increase, making the individual susceptible to colds and flu.

Cytokines comprise groups of proteins and peptides or even glycoproteins, produced by certain cells within the immune system. T-cells are produced within the thymus gland, and they influence how well a person responds to any challenges encountered by the immune system.

Dr. Balachandran is explicit about the role sleep deprivation plays in weakening a person's immune system, asserting that people in the habit of partying all night long reduce their capacity to fight not only colds but also infections caused by bacteria.

He also reiterates the importance of sleeping a minimum of seven hours a day, stating that sleeping for six hours and less hastens the individual's mortality.

In general, experts are in concurrence that whereas there are many reasons that lead to people falling ill, continued sleep deprivation increases the chances of catching a cold or developing other illnesses owing to a weakened immune system.

Some research findings involved eleven pairs of identical twins, whose patterns of sleep were monitored and recorded.

One of each twin slept shorter hours while the other slept the recommended number of hours of seven and over. When samples of blood were taken from them, it was found that the twins who slept shorter periods had their immune systems depressed while those of the others were unchanged.

As Dr. Nathaniel Watson of UW Medicine Sleep Center explains, people's immune systems function optimally when they have been getting sufficient sleep, where adequacy of sleep means a minimum of seven hours.

In the study involving twins, the researchers concluded that use of twins was preferable because the study did not have to cater for genetic differences in individuals, which are said to influence sleep patterns and durations to the extent of thirty one to fifty-five percent.

In support of the findings, Dr. Sina Gharib of UW Medicine's Computational Medicine Core cited results of laboratory experiments, which indicate that any time sleep is curtailed for a defined period inflammatory markers increase and end up activating the immune cells.

He explained it was evident that when people chronically slept for short durations, the programs associated with the individual's immune system response, and which are responsible for proper circulation of the white blood cells, shut down.

Like other experts, Dr. Watson underlines the fact that people who are consistently deprived of sleep respond poorly to vaccines, and says if exposed to the rhinovirus, for example, such people would have a higher chance of catching it due to the low response of their antibodies.

Reason Fevers Increase in the Night

It is a common observation that fevers tend to rise in the night, but as Dr. Balachandran observes, this only happens when the person is sleeping.

The reason is that this is the time the body is busy fighting any infection in the body, and if one does not sleep such infection is bound to weaken the person without any signal in form of a fever.

The doctor also makes an interesting observation, which is that the flu vaccine does not work well with people who are deprived of sleep; meaning, the vaccine does not offer them sufficient protection.

Another doctor, who is a pulmonologist dealing with sleep medicine, Dr. John Park, concurs, explaining that people who are deprived of sleep have suppressed immune responses, and they also produce less amount of antibodies in response to particular vaccines.

Dr. Park who is based in Rochester, Minnesota, says the body of a person deprived of sleep requires a bit of time before it can begin to respond to immunization, and so such a person may still become ill when exposed to the flu-causing virus while a person who enjoys good sleep is effectively protected by the vaccine.

Chapter 5: Insomnia and Degenerative Diseases

Experts seem to have found a link between insomnia and degenerative diseases, with insomnia sometimes being just a symptom and not a cause.

Fatal Familial Insomnia

Fatal Familial Insomnia, abbreviated as FFI, is a health disorder that affects the brain. It is genetic and degenerative. This disorder that is, nevertheless, rare, is marked by inability to fall asleep, which basically means insomnia.

In the beginning the problem is mild, but then it progressively becomes worse and leads to serious deterioration of both the physical health as well as the mental.

Sometimes the autonomic nervous system, or ANS, of someone with FFI becomes dysfunctional, and this adversely affects the person's daily life because the ANS is in charge of all involuntary processes of the body; those that happen automatically, such as breathing, regulation of body temperature and the like.

Origin and Symptoms of FFI

Different people with FFI manifest different symptoms depending on the specific area of the ANS the disorder has affected.

Although generally the cause of FFI is presence of some abnormal variant within the protein gene related to the prion, or PRPN for prion-related protein, there are people whose onset of the disease is just random. This latter case is referred to as SFI, or sporadic fatal insomnia.

The PRPN gene is responsible for producing a person's prion protein, and if this gene changes in any way, the prion protein generated is abnormal in shape.

Note that when the term 'prion protein' is used it means the same thing as simply 'prion'. The kind of abnormality in the prion is basically being misfolded, and the prion has been proven to introduce toxicity into the body.

In the condition of FFI, those prions that are abnormal accumulate in the thalamus of the person's brain, and this, in turn, causes the loss of neurons, which are nerve cells, in a progressive manner.

It is this same build-up of abnormal cells that causes the other different symptoms linked to FFI.

The progressive nature of FFI means it can begin when the person is in the middle age, and in some cases earlier or even later, with insomnia being evident.

At first the insomnia is mild, and it progresses until the person is left enjoying minimal sleep. Whatever stage in life insomnia sets in for people with FFI, it happens suddenly, and the disease progression can be rapid, incapacitating the person in a matter of months.

Sometimes the person with FFI manages to fall asleep, but every time the sleep is filled with dreams that are so vivid that they interfere with sleep. Soon, the person becomes physically and mentally unwell, and since a cure for the disease is yet to be found, FFI patients end up falling into coma and finally dying.

Another symptom of FFI is dementia, which sometimes manifests alongside insomnia. Just like insomnia, dementia in people with FFI is progressive, where the person's capacity to think and remember progressively worsens.

Other affected functions are those of cognition and language, as the person's general behavior changes for the worse.

There are also cases of FFI where signs are subtle and could easily be ignored. These are signs like forgetfulness, unplanned loss of weight, diminishing capacity to concentrate, and sometimes having problems with speech.

Also some people experience periods of confusion, while others have episodes of hallucination.

Other Symptoms of FFI

Apart from insomnia, dementia, and the other rather subtle symptoms of FFI, there are other disturbing ones that affect some individuals and they include the tendency to see things in double; a condition referred to as diplopia.

Another of these symptoms is having eye movements that are abnormal and jerky, a condition known as nystagmus.

There are still other symptoms associated with FFI, and they include dysphagia or difficulty in swallowing.

Dysarthria, which is a problem of slurring in speech, is another of FFI's symptoms.

Whichever of these symptoms individuals with FFI manifest, ultimately they end up having difficulty coordinating movements that they would otherwise do with ease; a condition known as ataxia.

Their movements are abnormal and twitchy, with evident tremors and muscle spasms that are jerky; a condition termed as myoclonus.

People whose FFI develops in this manner sometimes have symptoms close to those of Parkinson's disease.

FFI Symptoms that Affect the ANS
There are other symptoms people with FFI develop, and they interfere with the function of the autonomic nervous system.

These symptoms manifest variously among different people, the determinant factor being the section of the ANS the FFI has affected.

Some people become feverish while others develop tachycardia, which means their hearts beat abnormally fast; others develop hypertension or high blood pressure; or elevated levels of sweating otherwise known as hyperhidrosis.

The kind of sweating referred to as hyperhidrosis is confined to a specific area of the body as opposed to the body as a whole.

Other symptoms in this category include producing excessive tears, having constipation, becoming anxious or depressed, and some people even experience sexual dysfunction.

Frequency and Prevalence of FFI

It is not easy to determine the frequency of FFI because of its rarity, but it should be noted that the condition has been reported among populations across the globe.

It has been observed to affect both genders with equal measure, with the onset ranging from forty-five to fifty years of age. However, there are a few instances where people were noted to have developed FFI symptoms in their teenage or past the age of seventy.

Insomnia Related to Parkinson's disease

Parkinson's disease is among the degenerative diseases that affect a person's sleep. It is a health disorder that causes nerves to gradually stop working; hence the reason it is termed a neurodegenerative disorder.

As the disease sets in, the nerve cells within the brain that are responsible for production of dopamine begin to diminish.

It is important to note that dopamine is that molecule responsible for signaling cells, so that information is relayed among different cells of the nerves as well as between a person's brain and the various muscles of the body. In this capacity, dopamine is considered a neurotransmitter.

Parkinson's Symptoms that Affect the Motor System

When there is not sufficient amount of dopamine in the brain, the person begins to show symptoms affecting his/her motor system, which include tremors, rigidity and poor balance, as well as unusual slowness when making movements, otherwise termed bradykinesia.

Parkinson's Symptoms that affect the Non-Motor System

Insufficiency of dopamine has also been found to cause symptoms of a non-motor nature, among them challenges in sleeping. Other symptoms in this category include poor speech and cognition.

Nature of Sleep Problems linked to Parkinson's Disease

The sleep-related problems that people with Parkinson's disease encounter can be categorized into three: incapacity to fall asleep, challenges remaining asleep, and enjoying quality sleep where 'quality' denotes restful.

When people with Parkinson's have trouble falling asleep, it can be a result of varying symptoms.

Causes of Insomnia in Parkinson's Patients
Sometimes the Parkinson's patient may be on medication that has been helping him/her sleep well, but at some point the effect of the medication begins to wear off. This can make the symptoms of Parkinson's like rigidity or even tremors worsen; hence such a person is unable to resume sleep.

If this is found to be the case by the physician in charge, the patient's medication schedule can be adjusted so that the rate at which the medication clears from system does not affect the person.

In the case where the patient's sleep is disrupted by the ending of the medication effect, the doctor might prescribe for the patient a method where medication is delivered continuously, as exemplified by use of a patch.

Other times the doctor might choose to prescribe some sleep medication for the patient, all in an effort to fight insomnia.

The reason it is very important that insomnia be addressed in patients with Parkinson's disease is that it has been found to have a direct correlation with depression as far as people with Parkinson's are concerned.

There are several other problems associated with the Parkinson's disease that often lead to insomnia.

Sometimes even when the patients manage to fall asleep, the sleep ends up being fragmented; and this often interferes with the person's capacity to pay attention and even to think.

Among the factors that cause fragmented sleep in patients with Parkinson's is nocturia, which is the tendency to urinate very frequently. Others include hallucinations and experience of altered dreams.

Sleep Apnea in Parkinson's Patients
Sleep apnea is also a factor in patients of Parkinson's.

One research study was carried out to try and establish the connection between Parkinson's and sleep apnea, and it involved about three thousand two hundred subjects.

One hundred and ninety-four of those subjects had Parkinson's disease and seventy-seven had conditions almost similar to those of Parkinson's, and it was established that the prevalence of sleep apnea was higher in people who had Parkinson's than those who did not have the disease.

A different study established that prevalence of sleep apnea in patients with Parkinson's was higher in women than in men.

There was yet another observation made in a different study involving Parkinson's patients, which was that if the person's laryngopharynx is affected by motor dysfunction, then that person is likely to develop sleep apnea.

Note that the laryngopharynx is that part of the body that facilitates food passage as well as air passage to the throat.

In order to protect the patient from insomnia caused by sleep apnea, the doctor can prescribe the use of oral appliances, or devices that put pressure on the airway to maintain it open.

Such devices include CPAP or Continuous Positive Airway Pressure. Sometimes doctors suggest surgery where such devices fail to work, but such a move, like others of a medical nature, is determined on a case-by-case basis.

Insomnia Related to Alzheimer's disease

Alzheimer's disease is a medical disorder that leads to the cells of the brain wasting away or degenerating, and subsequently dying.

The disease is progressive, just like Parkinson's, and it has been found to be the greatest reason people develop dementia.

When people develop Alzheimer's, their capacity to think begins to decline, and all their skills – behavioral as well as social – begin to deteriorate.

This continuing incapacitation ends up disrupting the individual's capacity to be independent even on the most mundane of tasks. Worse still, the person begins to develop irregular patterns of sleep.

The reason for changes in sleep patterns has not been fully understood by experts, but they are believed to be the result of the negative effects of Alzheimer's on the person's brain.

Although serious changes in sleep patterns often develop in later phases of the illness, it has been observed they can also occur in the early stages.

Chapter 6: Natural Treatments of Insomnia

It has been established that having a section of the working population being sleep-deprived costs the country around sixty-three billion dollars every year, a cost incurred through loss of productivity.

Across the US, the estimated number of days lost every year in terms of productivity is two hundred and fifty-two million, because even though people do report to work as expected, for a big percentage, their efficiency is below par.

According to Professor Ronald C. Kessler of Harvard Medical School, sleep deprived Americans manage to report to work but they accomplish less than expected because they are exhausted.

The best way to overcome this problem is to find solutions to the root cause of the sleeping problem, and then begin to sleep better. Although there are different approaches to the problem, some are more appealing than others while others appear to be simpler. Among the simplest solutions is the use of medications.

Why Sleeping Pills Are Not the Best Solution

While taking sleeping pills succeeds in inducing sleep, the sleeping problem is only temporarily solved. Moreover, such medications often have unfavorable side effects such as headache and sore muscles.

Sometimes reliance on medications to fight insomnia makes people suffer constipation or dizziness, and other times they develop dry mouths, problems of concentration, and feeling of fatigue during the day.

For those who are lucky not to suffer such negative side effects, they often develop tolerance to the sleeping pills.

This means one has to take a higher dose in order to have the same effect as before, or the pills have no effect at all despite an increase in dosage.

For this reason, it is more preferable to try out solutions that are reasonably long lasting and with minimal side effects.

In fact, Dr. Stephen Winiarski, who notes that there are millions of people reliant on over-the-counter medications like Unisom, Lunesta and even Ambien, asserts that as long as these prescription medications help people fall asleep, they often ignore to establish the problem underlying the original problem of insomnia.

The doctor recommends trying out solutions that do not involve medication, because medications are only a temporary solution.

Non-medication Solutions to Insomnia

The environment within which you try to get sleep matters immensely. There are environments that are disruptive and others that are conducive to sleep.

Make Your Bedroom Sleep-friendly

Although often people take sleep deprivation as a stand-alone problem, some experts think it can lead to unwanted weight gain, and greater risk of developing diabetes and other chronic ailments.

In fact, Dr. Adnan Pervez who practices sleep medicine at REX Sleep Disorder Centre says it is important to consider sleep an essential component of life.

He notes that sleep covers a third of an individual's life, and it gives room for the body to restore itself so that one is able to function at daytime.

The doctor also points out that not only does the body rejuvenate during sleep, but its systems are able to regenerate even as hormonal adjustments take place. In fact, growth hormones are produced at night alongside the sleep-inducing hormone, melatonin.

One of the ways to encourage and enhance sleep without resorting to medication is making the bedroom conducive. In the next part of this chapter, you will learn what you can do to make your bedroom sleep friendly.

Clear distracting objects

Scientists believe people and animals can be conditioned to associate certain behavior or certain places with an event or activity. As far as the bedroom is concerned, it helps when you are able to associate it with sleep. That is why any time you plan on sleeping it is important that you go to the bedroom.

Nevertheless, this norm can be disrupted if you have some items in the room that grab your attention any time you enter. Disruptive sights can include a pile of work-related papers, gym equipment, computers, video games and the like.

Each one of them tends to draw your attention to the activity it is associated with and hence interferes with the natural process of falling asleep.

For that reason, you need to ensure all such objects are out of sight as you embark on sleep. Without them, your mind is bound to switch to rest mode relatively faster and ultimately fall asleep.

Keep your bedroom quiet

While you should not play loud music or have people talking in your bedroom as you try to fall asleep, you should also ensure the location of your bedroom does not absorb noise from outside.

If there are habitually disruptive noises from your neighbor's compound, such as dog barking or slamming of car doors late at night, ensure to select a room far from that end of the house to use as your bedroom.

If you have roommates, ask them to cooperate and keep the volume of the music system or TV down.

If you do not speak out your concerns you may end up getting upset, and building up frustration can only make you more agitated and anxious; which can only aggravate your sleeping problem.

Remember sleep deprivation is a societal problem and not one confined to a particular class of people. Hence, those who live in big residences can have disruptions just as much as those who live in apartments.

Use a White-noise Machine

In case there are still noise disruptions beyond your control, try to make use of earplugs or headphones to filter out such noises. You can also make use of some high-tech gadget known as 'white-noise machine' or a 'sound machine', which produces sounds that are so soothing that they promote relaxation and lead you to sleep.

Convenience of Sound Machines
Besides providing lullaby-like sounds, the white-
noise machines have the advantage of being
unobtrusive. The common ones are around four
inches in broadness with the height ranging
from two inches to below six inches.

These machines are also equipped with a variety
of sounds, and so you are able to choose your
favorite. For example, you can choose to listen to
the sounds of rainfall, of a blowing fan, ocean
waves, fascinating sounds of the night, and such
others.

Another advantage of using a sound machine to
invite sleep is that you are in control of the
sound volume. In case you want to drown some
irritating noise in the environment, you could
opt to make the machine sounds high, even up
to eighty-five decibels.

On the other hand, if you are in an environment
that is already quiet but you just want to
enhance the speed at which you fall asleep, you
may choose to tune the machine volume to a low
setting that is barely audible.

There is still another benefit sound machines have, and that is having a timer. Mostly they have a sixty-minute timer, which means you can set the number of minutes you want the machine to continue producing the soothing sounds.

It is important to note that although sound machines are helpful to adults as well as children, the American Academy of Pediatrics advises that any sound machine meant for use by a child should not exceed fifty decibels.

Also, the machine should not be any closer to the baby than two hundred centimeters.

Keep the Bedroom Dim

Bright light is a big distraction for someone getting ready to sleep, and even for someone who has already fallen asleep.

One big reason is that light has a way of naturally suppressing melatonin, a hormone related with regulating sleep.

As long as there is light in the bedroom, the mechanism of the body translates that to mean it is daytime and not time to sleep, and so the body does not produce the level of melatonin required for proper sleep.

That is the major reason people generally find themselves waking up at daybreak. The presence of light in their environment naturally signals the body that its daytime and you should be awake.

It needs to be noted that light has the same impact on sleep, whether it comes from the sun or from artificial sources like electricity bulbs.

Whenever possible, it is helpful to have a switch that allows the enabling for dimming lights, so that as you prepare to lie down to sleep you can dim the lights, and then once you are well set to sleep you can switch off the lights completely.

Such gradual dimming of your bedroom communicates to your body and mind that it is about time to go to sleep.

Leave Your Phone Alone

It is advisable to turn off your phone, or at least set it on airplane mode, before you go to bed, because then no in-coming call can interrupt your sleep.

For those whose nature of work demands that they be on call, they can have a separate phone or landline for communication.

The biggest problem with operating your phone when it is time for bed is that doing so puts your mind into active mode, at a time when you should be doing your best to relax so that you can doze off.

Moreover, the LCD screen of the phone is known for its emission of shortwave light that is blue in color, and as you operate your phone the light hits the eyes directly.

The sharp blue in that light communicates to the body's system that there is need to suppress melatonin; and with that any sleep you may have had begins to fade away.

For those who cherish the habit of reading something just before bedtime, it is recommended that they use e-readers that are non-LCD, because unlike phones, these do not

emit blue-colored light directly into the readers'
eyes.

Use Relaxing Colors for Bedroom

To calm your nerves and brain while in the
bedroom, decorate the room with calming
colors. Light blue or light green or even grey are
great for the bedroom in this respect. In contrast,
trying to sleep in a room painted with faux
graffiti or the entire rainbow spectrum running
zigzag would be too stimulating. As such, you
would be sabotaging your sleep process instead
of enhancing it.

Note that even singular sharp colors such as red
can be disruptive to the sleep process. They can
even cause elevated heart rate and blood
pressure, hence making the sleep situation even
worse.

In cases where the wall color is neither
commendable nor too bad, the appearance of the
room could be improved by using bedding with
sleep-friendly colors.

Some experts suggest a dusty blue or some light grey piece of bedding to be spread at the foot of the bed.

Above all, your bedroom should be clean even before you prepare to tidy it up and decorate it. The reason for this is that a clean environment helps to keep breathing problems away, but one that is dusty or smelly can cause blockage in the respiratory system that could lead to sleep apnea. It should be remembered that sleep apnea is a big factor in sleep interruptions.

Sleep Enhancing Fragrances

Alongside the change of bedroom ambience by giving it the appropriate lighting and color, the environment can still be improved by making use of some sleep enhancing fragrances. Those that are best for the bedroom causes you to relax, so that even if you had a tedious and hectic day you end up feeling relaxed both physically and mentally.

Sleep experts recommend fragrances such as lavender and jasmine, and even vanilla. Although the fragrances can be found in sprays and different air fresheners, essential oils are sometimes preferred when there is someone around with allergies. This is considered aromatherapy.

It is easier to select pure essential oils that are suitable for the person with allergies than it is to find a spray that is guaranteed not to cause irritation. The most convenient way to improve the bedroom environment using essential oils is to diffuse them using one of the diffusers available in the market.

Keep the Temperature Cool

Since the temperature of the body falls as you begin to fall asleep, it is appropriate that the environment within which you are sleeping has a matching temperature. In short, the temperature of your body and that of your environment should correspond for you to be comfortable enough to fall asleep.

It is recommended that the bedroom temperature be within the range of 66° and 68° Fahrenheit as you sleep. An extra warm bedroom normally has the effect of stimulating your body and mind, and the result is becoming more alert and awake as opposed to being relaxed and sleepy.

Keep off the clock

Sometimes people fall into the temptation of checking the time when sleep seems to be evasive, but counting the number of hours you have lost, or those you would benefit from if you could instantly fall asleep, does not help you fall asleep faster.

Instead, it is likely to make you anxious; and consequently, you end up losing any sense of sleep that may have been creeping in.

In fact, if you are convinced sleep is nowhere close as you lie in bed, it would be better for you to exit the bedroom, and probably do some breathing exercises to make you relax.

The reason you are not encouraged to continue lying in bed when you have failed to fall asleep is that you risk worrying about being sleep deprived, and no kind of worry is good for sleep. You get the best sleep when you are relaxed and stress free.

Use a Comfortable Pillow

It is important to use a pillow that is comfortable if you are to have restorative sleep. Worn-out pillows are one source of discomfort that disrupts sleep at odd hours, and once sleep is cut short by physical discomfort it sometimes becomes difficult to fall asleep again soon.

According to experts, a pillow ought to be replaced every one and a half years, not only because it is likely to begin discomfort from then onward, but because it is likely to have gathered allergens like dust mites, mold and even dead skin that can be irritating to the skin. Besides allergens are irritants that can also be a health hazard.

A good pillow is one that leaves the head lying neutral as opposed to either being elevated toward the ceiling or being put in a sloping position with the chin pointing downward.

Criteria for Choosing a Good Pillow

A good pillow is one that improves your comfort as you lie in bed and hence enhances your chances of sleeping more peacefully and for longer.

It has already been established that such restorative sleep helps rejuvenate your body's systems, and therefore the use of a good pillow not only helps enhance your mental state, but also your physical wellbeing.

The way to know if a particular pillow is good for you is by considering how you feel once you awake. If you feel stressed around your neck, shoulders or generally parts of your upper body, consider using a different kind of pillow.

Still, you can determine if a pillow is good for you by taking into account how you normally sleep; or the position you adopt as you sleep. That is normally the position you often find yourself in when you wake up.

If you are among the many people who are used to sleeping on their side, you should use a pillow that comfortably supports your head, the neck, the ear, as well as the shoulder.

For anyone whose normal sleeping position is on the back, a thinner pillow is more preferable, as it helps minimize stress in the neck area.

Those who sleep on their stomachs are best served by pillows of the thinnest size, as these manage to keep their spines straight in a healthy way, thus minimizing stress in their lower back area.

Pillows for People with Pre-existing Health Conditions

The kinds of conditions that would make it important for you to be particular about how you choose and use your pillow include GERD or Gastroesophageal Reflux Disease; and sleep apnea.

Pillows that Help with Acid Reflux Problem

The problem of acid reflux can keep one awake in the night, leading to the myriad of problems associated with sleep deprivation.

Fortunately, there is a type of pillow designed to help mitigate this problem of acid reflux, and it is known as the wedge pillow.

Experts who recommend this type of pillow reckon there are around fifteen million people in the US with this problem that manifests as heartburn, which often leads to further problems of apnea and insomnia.

Heartburn should be understood as a symptom of the bigger problem of acid reflux, which develops if juices of the stomach inadvertently flow back to the gut and enter the esophagus. It is when this problem becomes chronic that it is medically referred to as GERD.

According to Dr. Rajkumar Dasgupta of the University of Southern California, one should suspect GERD if he/she regularly experiences heartburn twice or three times in a week.

Dr. Dasgupta is a specialist in sleep and pulmonary problems, and he asserts that the recommended pillow helps by countering the effect of gravity.

This means a person lying on the back might have acid flowing backwards toward the esophagus, but once the wedge pillow is well positioned, the upper body is on a little incline that ensures the chest is well above the abdomen.

Hence the force of gravity keeps the acid trickling the right way, which is downwards.

It should be noted that although a good pillow would be helpful to people with the acid problem, it is important that a persistent problem of heartburn be investigated by a doctor because such acid could cause damage to esophageal tissue.

Worse still, Dr. Dasgupta explains, persistent incidences of acid reflux could be a sign of a bigger medical problem, particularly when they occur alongside the problem of anemia or vomiting, or even swallowing or unexplained loss of weight.

Pillows that Help with the Apnea Problem

People with the problem of apnea, which is that problem of interrupted breathing, can also reduce the problem by using wedge pillows.

These special pillows, which fall into different categories termed bed wedges, mattress wedges and the under mattress wedges, greatly reduce, and sometimes solve, this problem of OSA or obstructive sleep apnea.

The Mattress Wedge

Mattress wedges are wedges used to fill gaps that exist between the topmost part of the bed mattresses and the headboards. Nevertheless, for purposes of solving the problem of acid reflux, such a wedge is put under the person's mattress. The effect is to raise the plane on which the person is lying, so that it is at an elevation of four to eight inches; the level medical experts recommend.

The Bed Wedge

Bed wedges are short and narrow, and they are placed on the bed's top area. They have the effect of raising the person's upper body to a comfortable angle.

One advantage bed wedges have above mattress wedges is that they are smaller in size, and therefore relocating with them is easier.

Under Mattress Wedge

Under mattress wedges are placed beneath the mattress for the purpose of raising the bed, so that one can sleep comfortably. These wedges also serve the same purpose as the mattress wedges, which is to inhibit the back-flow of acid to cause acid reflux.

Another problem that these wedges reduce is sleep apnea. For some people, solving the problem of sleep apnea also eliminates the problem of acid reflux.

Note that although the level of bed or mattress elevation that makes people comfortable varies from one person to another, it has been established that many people find comfort when the elevation puts the head at between twenty and thirty degrees.

Dr. Steven Park who has authored 'Sleep Interrupted' explains that when a person snores, and especially if he/she has sleep apnea, the esophagus acts as a straw, sucking stuff from the stomach upwards.

Whatever the cause of the acid reflux, the main idea is to have the person's sphincter valve hindering the acid from passing through after being pushed from the stomach.

The Orthopedic Pillow

Sometimes people with serious sleep apnea and acid reflux issues require specially designed pillows that are "ergonomic", usually created by chiropractors.

The pillow has a headrest cavity that is cradled and also a well contoured neck ridge, which respectively serve as great support for the person's head as well as the neck.

In addition to solving the problem of apnea and acid reflux, the orthopedic pillow solves any problem the person may have had of neck soreness or soreness of the back. Compared to the other wedges, the orthopedic pillow is pricier, but its versatility is also greater.

Pillows that Reduce Back Pain

People who suffer pain in their back can reduce the problem by using special pillows that help maintain the natural position of the spine, neutrally without making it too bent or too straight.

Among the appropriate pillows are those with indentation within their middle part, the area that serves as the head's cradle.

Other suitable pillows are those whose edges are thick, because they have the effect of filling the hollow space between the person's skull and the top part of his/her back. This serves as great relief to that back area, as pressure is taken off the person's neck.

Control Humidity

The level of humidity, just like temperature, can affect how well you sleep. In areas that have high humidity levels, normal evaporation does not take place as would be normally expected, and so the air around remains with plenty of moisture in form of vapor.

As a consequence, the sweating process that is supposed to help your body cool is not as effective; and this becomes a source of physical discomfort. Such is the discomfort that makes it difficult to sleep continuously for long periods particularly in areas that are hot and humid.

In addition to the physical discomfort occasioned by humidity, there are also the problems associated with dampness, as surfaces often become damp as humidity increases. Molds can grow as a result, and these bring their own health issues like fungal infections or even allergies.

The discomfort that these problems cause can easily interfere with normal sleep patterns and hence the quality of restorative sleep. Finding both a mattress and pillow products that are anti-fungal and anti-bacterial would be a good idea.

How to Deal with Dampness

Air conditioners are suitable for clearing dampness in the room, and you only need to run one for a couple of hours in a day for the air within to become drier.

If the environment in your bedroom is cool enough to make you comfortable just before bedtime, you have a better chance of falling asleep soundly with the body continuing its normal role of temperature regulation.

You do not need to run an air conditioner for the entire night. Where AC or air conditioning system is not available, a fan can help enhance the flow of air within the room; and a dehumidifier can help suck out the dampness.

How to Deal with too much Dryness

Even though humidity can interfere with one's ability to sustain sleep, a little of it is required in order to avoid the problem of dry nasal passage, cracking of lips or even sneezing. In fact, when the air is too dry, some forms of colds tend to increase alongside other viral ailments.

Ailments aside, the respiratory system needs to be well lubricated in order to function properly, and dryness that emanates from too little humidity often leads to irritation of the throat or a feeling of being gagged, developments that make it difficult to sleep.

Ways to raise Humidity Level

There are humidifiers in the market that can help to increase the level of humidity in the house, especially in the bedroom.

Note the importance of ensuring the water used in the humidifier is distilled because once water that has impurities has settled in the small reservoir for a while, bacteria can begin to develop alongside allergens.

In fact, the water in the humidifier ought to be replaced regularly, and the equipment cleaned in three-day intervals. Note that it is fine to leave the humidifier running as you sleep.

How to Assess Humidity Level

In case you are unsure when you need to increase humidity or when to decrease it, you can make use of a hygrometer, a gadget that measures humidity levels.

A simple one in the form of a sling psychrometer is good enough. This one comprises two adjoined thermometers, one of them a normal thermometer and the other one a wet-bulb thermometer.

The recommended humidity is from thirty to fifty percent, the range within which breathing is easy and not strained. You can also opt to buy a humidifier that already has a built-in hygrometer.

Among the remedies suggested for insomnia, some are more suitable to some people than others, all depending on the root cause of the problem. For some people, poor sleep could just be the result of continuous travel in the recent past (time zone related), a problem that may be better solved with regular warm showers and aromatherapy.

This means it is crucial that every person tries to establish the reason their sleep is not optimal, to ensure the solution being applied is appropriate.

Whenever there is no obvious reason for the problem, one ought to consult a medical practitioner for professional advice.

In the meantime, it would help to establish a daily routine that enables you to begin relaxing as evening approaches. This means doing away with strenuous and mind challenging activities earlier in the day, in preparation for a night of relaxation.

Chapter 7: Adopting Sleep-Enhancing Behavior

One way of ensuring you do not suffer anxiety is to be in control of what happens in your life. This should begin with the things you engage in on a day-to-day basis, and the timing you give those activities.

This means it is important to have a lifestyle that is well structured, and to adhere to your well thought out plan.

Lifestyle Behavior that Enhances Quality of Sleep

Whereas some problems like those associated with disease may be beyond your control, there are still some lifestyle adjustments that one can make to mitigate sleep-related problems.

Exercising

An individual who is physically active is likely to enjoy better sleep than one who leads a sedentary lifestyle.

In fact, there is a study that has shown that people who exercise a minimum of one hour per day in five days of the week have better quality sleep in the REM phase than those who do not.

Nevertheless, the good news is that even exercising for half an hour on a regular basis of three or even four days in a week still have better quality sleep than people who hardly exercise.

As for the timing, experts reckon morning exercises produce better results than exercises done any other time of the day, although they have not been able to explain the reason.

Timing notwithstanding, the important point to note is that exercising has several benefits that lead to improved sleep; like relaxation and reduced levels of anxiety or depression. Another great benefit of regular exercise is maintenance of the normal sleep-wake cycle.

Exposure to Sunlight

Even in locations where the sun does not shine bright, exposing yourself to periods of sunlight can enhance the body's production of melatonin the natural way.

A body that absorbs sufficient sunlight is able to synchronize its inner clock with the times of the day, so that it produces the different hormones at their appropriate times.

For example, hormones that boost energy are released in the day while those like melatonin that cause relaxation and induce sleep are produced after dusk.

An expert from the Parrish Sleep Disorder Center, Michele Roberge, who is also a neuro-diagnostic technologist, explains that light has a way of triggering production of signals by the pineal gland, which then causes the release of wake-enhancing hormones.

Roberge underscores the importance of exposing yourself to sunlight, saying that even walking to collect mail from outside the house on a regular basis in the morning can be beneficial to a person with insomnia.

As is explained by sleep experts, you will get your body well tuned to embrace sleep at appropriate times and ditch it at the right time if you get into the habit of letting plenty of light into your house once you have woken up.

This sends a clear message to your body's system that time to be alert has arrived. It is recommended that your keep your environment well lit throughout the day, and if the inside is not well-lit sitting beside an open window that has sunlight coming through would be helpful.

Whenever possible, spend some time outside even if it means utilizing part of your lunch break for that. Experts have observed that doing so often increases your sleeping time by an hour or so at night.

Keeping Stress under Check

There are some measures you can take in addition to morning or daytime exercise, to minimize stress levels so that you are mentally in shape for sleep when night comes.

Shifting your mind from high activity

Make it a habit to stop engaging in stimulating activities an hour prior to bedtime; or half an hour before at the minimum.

In today's context, this includes avoiding texting on smart phones and abandoning work-related activities.

If watching television, choose calming programs as opposed to those that cause you tension.

You can also tune into some pleasant calming music even before you enter the bedroom, so that you can begin transitioning to the required state of relaxation conducive to sleep.

There are also some breathing exercises that are good at calming both the body and the brain, and they include taking in a number of deep breaths.

In fact, such a breathing routine decompresses your system and also reduces your heart rate as well as blood pressure. This leaves you relaxed and calm.

Practicing Journaling

The purpose of journaling is to ensure you have prepared your system to stop disruptive thoughts.

You need to set aside any thoughts that make you extra alert when you are supposed to be putting your mind to rest.

Even if the thoughts are not disturbing but they are leading your mind to think critically, they are still bound to delay the onset of sleep.

One way of getting your mind to adhere to your wishes of eliminating serious thoughts is by scribbling down, termed 'journaling', the serious issues you want to address in the week or even the following day; and this is best done sometime during the afternoon.

That will put your mind at rest and the pending issues will not keep erupting in your mind at night.

With thought provoking issues out of the way, be open to embracing pleasant thoughts, because those are great at enhancing your state of relaxation that you want in preparation for sleep.

It was reported in 'Applied Psychology' sometime ago that some students who maintained a journal to write their daily experiences that they were grateful for, and spent a quarter of an hour every night making their entries, had little or no worries at bedtime. Hence, they slept better.

Practicing progressive muscle relaxation
This is a simple exercise where you are required to tense and relax your toes in alternate turns.

Sleep disorder experts from the medical center at the University of Maryland recommend doing this exercise long enough to count up to ten.

The effect of the exercise is to relieve any energy that may have been pent up, and as a result having a wave of relaxation set in.

Retiring to Bed Early

When you go to bed early, any thoughts occupying your mind are likely to disappear before long.

On the contrary, once you take long to go to bed you give room for thoughts to occupy your mind.

As one study has shown, this is a good time for negative thoughts to flood your mind, and often they are overwhelming enough to interfere with your sleep.

Adopt a Sleep-friendly Diet

While the general recommendation is to feed on a balanced diet, there are certain foods that are known to sabotage sleep especially when consumed at the end of the day.

On the other hand, some foods are great at enhancing sleep, often because they have a calming effect.

It is for that reason that experts recommend incorporating one or more of the sleep enhancing foods in your evening meal, whether to be part of the main dinner or to snack on before bed, while avoiding foods that tend to be disruptive to sleep.

Sleep-enhancing Foods

Cheese and Almonds

Cheese is considered suitable for your evening as it relaxes your body to the extent of making you sleepy.

The reason for this effect is that cheese has plenty of tryptophan, a kind of amino acid credited with production of serotonin, which is a neurotransmitter that relaxes the body and induces sleep.

As for almonds or other crunchy nuts, they are not only rich in tryptophan, but they are also rich in calcium as well as magnesium.

Both of these minerals are great at enhancing the quality of sleep.

Salmon and Other Omega-3 Rich Foods

Meals rich in Omega-3 fats and particularly DHA are known to enhance sleep. DHA stands for docosahexaenoic acid, one of the three fatty acids contained in Omega-3.

DHA-rich foods include seafood like salmon, halibut, mackerel as well as tuna and herring; edible algae; as well as eggs.

One report of a British study carried by the Journal of Sleep Research indicated that foods rich in this Omega-3 fatty acid DHA are great at nurturing sleep.

Cherries

The reason cherries are recommended as a component of your evening meal is that they contain melatonin, a hormone that has been proven to be effective in enhancing sleep. You can make it your dessert after dinner, whether freshly picked, from your freezer after thawing, or even in the form of juice.

A report carried by the Journal of the Federation of American Societies for Experimental Biology indicated that individuals who drank two glasses of tart cherry juice every night enjoyed one and a half extra hours of sleep, compared to the period before the routine started.

Milk with low percentage of fat

One of the reasons milk is recommended as part of your evening meal is that it is rich in calcium, one of the minerals known to enhance production of melatonin.

Another reason is that it is good at reducing chances of developing acid reflux, hence countering heartburn that is a big factor in sleep disruption.

Ripe Bananas

The benefits of ripe bananas in enhancing sleep which emanates from the fact that they contain a significant level of magnesium and potassium; minerals great at promoting relaxation of the muscles.

Ripe bananas also contain tryptophan that is known to enhance sleep.

Foods Disruptive to Sleep

Even as you feed on sleep enhancing foods, you should also steer clear of foods that have a negative effect on either your sleeping pattern or the quality of your sleep.

Caffeine sabotages sleep

Foods with caffeine are not good for sleep.

According to Dr. Jaques, a senior research scientist, caffeine has a way of binding the adenosine receptors in the brain, thus inhibiting the capacity of the compound called adenosine to bind them as it normally does.

Whereas without caffeine the binding of the adenosine receptors leads to reduced neural activity and promotion of sleepiness, the effect of caffeine is to counter the slowing down of neural activity.

The sleepy effect is actually countered by the stimulation effect of caffeine on the CNS or central nervous system.

Dr. Ian Dunican who is a sleep expert confirms that caffeine is responsible for delayed onset of sleep, and says it can also cause sleep interruptions even after you have managed to fall asleep.

The reason for this as Dunican's explanation is that caffeine takes one hour to reach its peak effect once you have consumed it and remains active in the body for an entire eight hours and sometimes longer.

Common foods that have significant amounts of caffeine, according to Dr. Marta Maczaj of Port Jefferson's St. Charles Sleep Disorders Center, include coffee, black tea and green tea, as well as chocolate, energy drinks and soda.

Dr. Maczaj advises those whose like caffeinated foods to ensure they limit their consumption to noon; but for those who still have problems sleeping, total consumption of such foods should be more restricted or totally curtailed.

The explanation given by Dr. Amy Bender, a senior research scientist whose specialty is sleep performance, is that not only does caffeine have an arousal effect, but it makes sleep latency longer.

As such, falling asleep takes longer than normal, and chances of sleep being disrupted thereafter are raised due to caffeine's tendency to increase the activity of the brain waves.

Avoid Spicy Foods for Dinner

Foods that are spicy have been found to interfere with the richness of sleep, but there is not yet scientific evidence to explain the reason.

Some experts suspect it could have something to do with the effect spicy foods like sriracha and mustard tend to have on body temperature, raising it to levels above normal.

The negative impact of spicy foods on sleep has been documented in the International Journal of Psychophysiology, where it is said that because of the spices, people take longer to fall asleep and end up not enjoying quality sleep.

Minimize fatty foods

According to the National Sleep Foundation, people who consume foods that are high in fat end up sleeping less than those who consume less fatty foods.

Experts suspect the reason is the strain that grease puts on the digestive function, making the person significantly uncomfortable and therefore not relaxed enough to have a good night's sleep.

Chapter 8: Herbal Remedies versus OTC Drugs

There are herbs that can be taken plainly or in foodstuff for the purpose of alleviating the sleep problem.

Nevertheless, experts insist that consuming sleep-friendly products is not a substitute for a favorable sleep regimen, but it can complement it.

Apart from the herbs already in use for culinary purposes, it is always advisable to discuss with the doctor about your intent to consume others as sleep enhancers, just like you should before beginning to rely on sleep medications.

Such discussions are even more pertinent in cases where people are on medication for other ailments, as there may be some fatal interactions.

Herbal Remedies

Chamomile

Chamomile is a herb mostly taken as tea, which people find delicious and relaxing. It has, in fact, been found to calm nerves and to minimize anxiety.

Owing mostly to its sedative effect, albeit mild, it serves well to mitigate insomnia. For best effect in enhancing sleep, two or three tea bags per evening are recommended.

St. John's Wort

St. John Wort is a yellow flower with a look of a weed, and it is good at easing symptoms of depression such as anxiety; consequently, keeping insomnia at bay.

It produces a tasty beverage once steeped, and so you can make it your evening beverage a while before bedtime.

However, the herb needs to be stored away from sunrays because once it is exposed it is affected by the UV rays in a way that makes it irritating to your skin.

The Valerian

The valerian root is another herb that makes a tea-like beverage just like chamomile.

For this one, it is the root that is effective in matters of insomnia treatment, as it eases anxiety and promotes relaxation.

Using a valerian drink in the night helps you catch sleep faster and remain asleep longer without interruptions.

Nevertheless, its use should not be long-term as scientists have reported some serious side effects.

The Kava Root

People within the Pacific islands have for long relied on the Kava root for relaxation, but although preliminary scientific findings have confirmed it is better than over-the-counter medications in the treatment of insomnia, it should be used with breaks and not over continuous long periods.

Scientists have their reservations about its impact on the liver if used for a long period.

Passionflower

One teaspoon of this tropical passionflower is normally boiled in water for around ten minutes, and after drinking it you do not take long before you begin to doze off. This herbal product has a mild sedating effect.

Melatonin

Although the body produces its own melatonin, you can still take melatonin supplements made from herbal extracts to regulate a distorted sleep pattern, and to enhance the quality of your sleep. Melatonin's role in the body is to induce sleep. It should be remembered that melatonin plays a central role in regulating a person's circadian rhythm.

The California poppy

This herb is so effective in inducing sleep that its drink needs to be taken just a short while before bedtime. Its preparation involves steeping the plant's leaves in hot water, where you leave them for around ten minutes.

The drink from these leaves that are a bright orange in color is known for easing anxiety and having a relaxing effect on the body as a whole.

It needs to be noted that even with all the goodness of herbal products in lessening insomnia, one still needs to be cautious about being over-reliant on them.

Any problem of insomnia that does not disappear for months on end should be referred to a doctor.

Alternatively, if you know the underlying non-medical reasons for the problem, you need to address them as a matter of priority.

In fact, to ensure there is little need for you to be entirely and continually dependent on herbal extracts and supplements in solving the problem of insomnia, you need to couple them with lifestyle changes like those already recommended in the book.

Sleeping Pills

The term 'sleeping pills' is generically used in reference to OTC-medication and prescription drugs, both of which help people with sleeping problems to fall asleep or remain asleep for a reasonable time.

Sometimes people refer to sleeping pills as hypnotics, and that is because of their capacity to induce sleep. The word, 'hypnotics', is derived from the Greek word 'hynos', which means 'sleep'.

Other times people refer to sleeping pills as sedatives, and that is because they have a calming effect that is so great that it causes drowsiness.

Sleeping pills have become popular over the years because they seem to solve sleep problems instantly. It is estimated that four percent of adults in the US use prescription sleeping pills due to sleep deprivation. Those who rely on over-the-counter sleeping pills range from three percent to eleven percent.

Benefits of Sleeping Pills

While most people take sleeping pills to initiate restorative sleep or to sleep longer on a normal night, others take them to help them go through certain uncomfortable situations.

For example, some people are unable to sleep when on a flight, and when the distance is long it means arriving at the destination feeling haggard and sometimes disoriented.

Although many people are able to overcome the sleep problem by use of headphones that cancel out noises, others find it difficult to catch sleep even when the plane is quiet and the flight is smooth. Those are the ones that Dr. Aneesa Das from Ohio State University says can justifiably make use of sleeping pills – not those on short-distance flights.

Categories of Sleeping Pills

There are different categories of sleeping pills, some of which contain a neurotransmitter referred to as GABA, which has the effect of reducing the brain's excitability.

GABA is an acronym for Gamma aminobutyric acid, an amino acid that inhibits particular signals of the brain thereby decreasing the activity in the nervous system. In fact, it is the very reason drugs like benzodiazepine are prescribed to ease anxiety.

OTC Medications

OTC medications are those that one can buy from a pharmacy without presenting a doctor's prescription, and some people like them because picking their choice of drug makes them feel in control of their wellbeing.

Using OTC medication is also less costly than using a prescription from a doctor, because the latter requires that you pay consultancy fees in most countries. Nevertheless, the use of OTC drugs is only worthwhile if medication is taken in the right dosage for the appropriate duration. Otherwise they can turn lethal.

It is even better if the pharmacy has qualified personnel to guide the buyers, so that they do not buy medications that can interact with others they may be already taking.

Among the commonly used OTC medications are melatonin and sedating antihistamines.

Melatonin

Melatonin is available in form of supplements, which function in a similar manner as the natural melatonin the body produces from the pineal gland as a hormone.

These supplements help to support the natural melatonin in regulating the circadian rhythm, so that one falls asleep and awakes at the right times.

Sedatives

The other common OTC medication type comprises the antihistamines with sedating effect.

Among the popular brands are Benadryl, Zzzquil and Unisom whose active ingredient is the antihistamine, diphenhyramine; Sominex whose active ingredient is promethazinen hydrochloride; and Doxylamine that is often taken to ease symptoms of common cold.

Prescription Sleeping Medications

Many of the prescription drugs are either benzodiazepines, whose active ingredient is diazepam, or the z-drugs whose active ingredients is one of three drugs with names beginning with 'z' – zolpidem, zaleplon or zopiclone.

One of the commonest prescription medicines for insomnia is Zolpidem, a z-drug, whose power comes from enhancing the effectiveness of GABA, the neurotransmitter that makes the brain less excitable. As a brand, it is known as 'Ambien'.

Zeleplon, another of the z-drugs, has 'Sonata' as its brand name, and is also in common use for insomnia.

Another z-drug used for insomnia is eszopiclone that goes by the brand name 'Lunesta'.

Temazepam falls under the group of benzodiazepines, and it goes by the brand name 'Restoril'.

Trazodone, whose active ingredient is trazodone hydrochloride, goes by the brand name 'Desyrel', and it is fundamentally an anti-depressant. Nevertheless, it is prescribed under the sedative-hypnotic kind of drugs to alleviate insomnia.

Disadvantages of Sleeping Pills

Countering sleep problems with medicines should be an occasional intervention but not a long-term remedy.

Many of the over-the-counter medications have antihistamines, and if used continuously people usually develop tolerance to them. This means the medication's sleep enhancing quality diminishes over time.

According to Dr.William Dement from Stanford University's sleep disorders clinic, chronic utilization of sleeping pills is not medically justifiable.

His remarks came as he expressed his concurrence with a 1992 article in the Mature Outlook magazine, which indicated that continued use of sleeping pills adversely affects a person's deep sleep and makes sleep less restorative.

He mentioned that the longest he personally prescribed sleeping pills for a patient was ten days, but mostly he kept it at one or two nights.

According to researchers, insomnia is merely a symptom and not the actual illness, and so the underlying problem should be sought and addressed instead of suppressing it with sleeping pills.

Another major problem with sleeping pills is their addictive nature. With long-term use, people tend to become dependent on them, so that they cannot sleep without taking them, and in the meantime can become edgy.

Although different pills may have different effects after long-term use, there are those effects that manifest in the short-term for many of them.

One of them is feeling drowsy during the day, even after a night of enhanced sleep. Others include having a dry mouth; feeling dizzy; developing a headache; suffering loss of memory; and finding it a problem to remain alert.

The side effects of pills like Diphenhydramine and Doxylamine, for example, include dry mouth; constipation; blurriness of vision; unusual retention of urine; and feeling of drowsiness during the day.

With Zolpidem, its most common side effects include dizziness, grogginess and fatigue, as well as diarrhea and headache.

However, in rare cases, people develop grave side effects like pre-existing depression they had becoming more aggravated; being agitated or anxious; developing confusion or aggression; having hallucinations; and worst of all having suicidal thoughts.

For medications like Lunesta, Halcion, Sonata, and even Ambien and Rozerem, additional side effects may be observed, such as tingling in the limbs or a burning sensation. Some people have also reported losing appetite or feeling generally weak the following day.

Other known side effects of sleeping pills include interference with proper breathing, especially for people who suffer from asthma and other respiratory problems. On the overall, anyone with a chronic lung-related problem like emphysema or any other chronic obstructive pulmonary disease should consider sleeping pills dangerous.

Emphysema is a lung condition where the air sacs are so damaged that they cause shortness of breath.

Other risky behavior that may not be necessarily fatal include dependency, which is sometimes psychological and other times physical. Even OTC medications can lead to such dependency, not just the prescription drugs.

Among the prescription medications known to cause dependency and addiction are barbiturates and Benzodiazepines, otherwise referred to as BZDs, BDZs, or even BZs. As such, one should avoid taking them on a daily basis or for extended periods.

Barbiturates are made out of barbiturate acid, and their main target is the central nervous system where they depress the nerves and relax the muscles. They also interfere with the GABA activity.

Although barbiturates are often used as anesthesia, it is good to know the ones commonly used, in case one gets prescribed some for insomnia.

The commonest within the US are amobarbital, butabarbital, pentobarbital, secobarbital, and belladonna plus phenobarbital, whose brand names are Amytal, Butisol, Nembutal, Seconal, and Donnatal.

While the side effects of melatonin are mild, there is still a chance of developing some headache, and feeling sleepy during the day.

There is also the problem of some OTC sleeping medications making you feel groggy and generally unwell the following day, a state commonly referred to as 'hangover effect'.

People also need to be aware that there are several sleep enhancing medications whose exact interactions are unknown even to medical professionals, and so even as they are used for their effectiveness, such use should be done with caution.

The Sleepwalking Side Effect

Sleepwalking, which is medically termed somnambulism, is among the most serious problems some sleeping pills cause.

Somnambulism is marked by a person getting up and beginning to walk without realizing it, and it happens after the person has been asleep for some time; and as the person is about to emerge from deep sleep.

If the person sleepwalking ends up resuming sleep without interference, he/she often retains no memory of such an episode. There are times when people talk incoherently as they sleepwalk, but they are not in a position to respond when spoken to.

Although sleepwalking sometimes runs in the family, some people's sleepwalking behavior is entirely ignited by sleeping pills. Sleepwalking is considered dangerous because there is no limit to the actions a person can engage in unconsciously, including some that are either complex or unsafe.

It is for this reason that the FDA demanded the use of a 'black box' alert or warning, to draw the attention of potential users to possible danger if they were to take the medication. Some of the risky behaviors linked to sleepwalking include drowning, causing accident while driving, or consuming lethal substances.

People who sleepwalk are said to have parasomnia, which is a sleep-related disorder that is marked by abnormal or unusual behavior. Owing to the risk posed by sleepwalking to self and other people, one may wish to avoid OTC medications that often have the side effect; like the diphenhydramines.

The Sleep-eating Side Effect

One of the disturbing side effects of sleeping pills is sleep-eating, which indicates the individual has parasomnia, a condition that affects the nervous system in a manner to cause abnormal behavior.

The other commonly known behavior under parasomnia is sleepwalking, which, like sleep-eating, is caused by the sleep medication, Ambien. Sleep-eating is sometimes referred to in short as SRED, which stands for 'Sleep Related Eating Disorder'.

According to Dr. Aris Latridis of Piedmont Healthcare and who specializes in sleep medicine, people with the sleep-eating disorder wake up at night and proceed to binge on food or even drink, but they have little or no recollection of that incident when they wake up in the morning.

It has been found that people with the condition usually wake up when in the non-REM phase of sleep, when sleep is at its deepest; the same phase sleepwalking manifests in some people.

The American Academy of Sleep Medicine has established that sleep-eating affects people whose age is in the range of 22yrs to 29yrs, and that the female gender are more susceptible than the male.

According to Dr. Latridis, the problem of sleep-eating is initiated by sleeping pills, the most notorious being Ambien, whose generic name is Zolpidem. Nevertheless, the doctor also says that other sleep medications like Halcion and other benzodiazepines can also cause sleep-eating.

While sleep-eating may not appear particularly dangerous, the fact that the night feeding is not triggered by hunger or thirst often leads to the individual gaining unwanted weight. Coupled with the fact that the behavior is beyond the person's control, the individual can also easily become depressed.

Another concern is the speed at which the entire episode of parasomnia takes place; ten minutes only, inclusive of the walk to and from the kitchen, and the feeding itself.

This means food may not be properly chewed. It also means that food requiring proper heating may not be done well. There is also the risk of the person hurting himself/herself through cuts or burns, or causing a fire in the premises.

It is also feared that the person experiencing this disorder may consume something not fit for human consumption, as his/her mind is still not alert or aware at the time.

How to Deal with Sleep-eating

It may appear easy to solve sleep-eating by simply locking away all food and drinks before going to bed, but according to Dr. Latridis, it is better to investigate what the actual trigger is, with a view to alleviating it. In case it is some medication causing the sleep-eating, the doctor reckons it can be substituted for another one, or you can simply be weaned off the medication.

Some medicines have also been known to alleviate sleep-eating, like Prozac, the anti-depressant. Other means of fighting off sleep-eating include behavior that reduces stress, and a favorable sleeping habit.

Insomnia Pills during Pregnancy
Sometimes pregnant women develop insomnia, and mostly that happens during the third trimester.

It is estimated that three quarters of pregnant women suffer insomnia during this period, although for some the problem of insomnia begins in the second trimester.

Usually insomnia increases the more other symptoms of pregnancy manifest, and as the increase in belly size makes it more difficult to lie comfortably in bed.

While insomnia on its own does not pose any serious risk to the mother or the unborn baby, it has the same negative effects to a pregnant woman as it has on anyone else; like experiencing fatigue during the day.

Nevertheless, worrying about insomnia can aggravate the situation and make catching sleep even more difficult, and so one should consider how best to enhance sleep rather than worrying about its deficiency.

In order to determine the best remedy for insomnia when pregnant, it is best to first consider what is interfering with sleep in the first place.

Often it is a combination of factors that can include hormonal change; leg cramps; frequent urge to empty the bladder; heartburn associated with pregnancy; increased body temperature caused by heightened rate of metabolism; pre-delivery anxiety; and such other pregnancy related issues.

How to Deal with Pregnancy-linked Insomnia

Many of the general recommendations made for the sake of improving the quality of sleep are also applicable to pregnant women.

In addition, when as a pregnant woman you get into bed and fail to fall asleep within half an hour, it may help to get up and engage in some light mental work, which is bound to challenge your mind; like paying your bills or preparing a grocery list for the next time you go out shopping.

Avoid counting the hours you have been awake or asleep, and instead focus on how you feel when you wake up. Sometimes you will feel relaxed even without clocking a full seven or eight hours.

Address any anxieties you have with someone like your spouse, because once they are sorted out you can enjoy peaceful uninterrupted sleep for the duration of your pregnancy. Examples of anxieties that can keep a pregnant woman awake include the kind of healthcare services available during delivery and health insurance coverage.

Other good ways of releasing anxiety or worries is writing down the persistent thoughts as they come to mind, or getting into the habit of meditating.

It is also helpful to get into a healthy eating habit, which includes avoiding caffeinated beverages and chocolate. These are particularly detrimental to sleep if consumed in the late hours of the afternoon or in the evening.

Part of the good eating habit is having dinner early in the evening, because feeding late means having the feeling of fullness as you go to bed, which may interfere with your falling or remaining asleep. Also, eating late night makes your body work more with processing food and digestion, when it should be repairing, restoring and regenerating other systems of the body.

Still on the issue of eating, it is advisable to maintain a reasonable eating pace; ensuring food is well chewed and swallowed without hurry. The importance of consuming dinner in this manner lies in avoiding heartburn, which often keeps one awake and tossing in bed.

While drinking plenty of fluids is advisable, it is best to fill the day's fluid requirement early in the evening as opposed to drinking late into the night, because it cuts down on the need to empty the bladder at night.

While engaging in heavy exercise near bedtime is discouraged, pregnant women need to do a bit of exercising every day, as that makes them sleepier as the night wears on. On the other hand, the aftermath of heavy exercise during the night would keep one awake long after the workout.

Another behavior pattern that can help you sleep at your chosen time and remain asleep till morning is developing some routine for going to bed. This means going to bed at the same hour every single day, and getting out of bed at the same time all days.

It also helps to have a preferred playlist of soothing songs that you can play at bedtime. For those who enjoy it, yoga routines that are considered serene can also help to keep off insomnia. Another alternative is having a warm bath before getting into bed.

Safe use of Sleeping Pills when Pregnant

Sleeping pills ought not to be used by anyone unless it is necessary to do so, and this stance is more pertinent for pregnant women. In fact, anyone pregnant should avoid self-medicating, and instead obtain a prescription from a medical doctor.

Nevertheless, some sleeping pills have been found to be relatively safe for pregnant women, and they include Unisom, Lunesta and Tylenol PM, as well as Sominex, Ambien and even Nytol.

There are also times when doctors recommend magnesium supplements as a means to deal with leg cramps or even constipation, and in such cases it is best to take the supplements at night because their muscle-relaxing capacity can help to lull you into sleep.

Safe Use of OTC Medication

Before contemplating using OTC medication, see if you can first discuss the issue with your physician.

The reason is that the professional knows the medications that interact with others, how any underlying condition you have might be aggravated, the duration within which you can optimally use the medications, and also the dosage appropriate for you.

However, if you decide to personally buy OTC medications, be careful with your selection so that you do not pick medications with potential to interact with other medications you are using. It may even be helpful to seek the opinion of the pharmacist selling you the sleeping pills.

For example, drugs like diphenhydramine and doxylamine are discouraged for anyone with asthma or any COPD, serious liver condition, closed-angle glaucoma, and obstruction of the digestive system.

Avoid OTC sleep medications if you are pregnant or even breastfeeding, or ensure you visit a doctor first and consult about your situation.

Only a doctor can ascertain if it is safe for a particular person to take a sleeping pill when pregnant, and which exact pill that would be and when to be taken.

The same case applies to people aged 75 years and above, because people at this age are at high risk of stroke and such other illnesses like dementia, which can be exacerbated by the effect of sleeping pills.

If it becomes necessary, use sleeping pills to temporarily solve your sleeping problem, but seek other means of alleviating the root problem in the long-term. Fourteen days is the longest anyone should be taking sleeping pills, beyond which the risk of dependency and other side effects becomes a real threat.

Avoid taking alcohol when using sleeping pills or any other form of sedative, because that would mean increasing the degree of sedation to dangerous levels. In fact, such sedation is often as bad as interaction of sleep medication with other medications, with potential to be fatal.

Also, when it comes to the tasks you undertake, ensure you avoid those that require you to be alert, because sleep medications interfere with mind alertness. Activities like driving or operating machinery should, therefore, be avoided, because they can be dangerous for you and others around.

Summary: Essence of Sleep and Alleviation of Sleep Disorders

Quality sleep is crucial to overall health, and more so for one to carry out the day-to-day activities in a normal manner. In fact, it is as important as a good feeding habit, because failure to adhere to either of them brings about disease and a state of depression that inhibit one's capacity to function normally.

According to Dr. Eva Selhub whose publications have appeared in Harvard Health Publishing of the Harvard Medical School, serotonin, the neurotransmitter from the gastrointestinal tract, not only regulates a person's mood, it also regulates appetite as well as sleep.

For the body to produce this chemical in the right amounts, one needs to consume foods with the amino acid, tryptophan, found in seeds and protein-rich foods like eggs and salmon, and vegetables like spinach.

One also needs to develop a daily routine that does not jeopardize chances of a good night's sleep. This means doing away with eating and drinking well before bedtime and finishing up mentally stimulating activities just as early.

It also means engaging in sleep enhancing activities as bedtime approaches, like serene yoga, taking a warm bath, or listening to soothing music.

It is also important that one addresses existing health conditions before they begin to have adverse effects on sleep; like having migraines investigated and treated, and any other health problem like skin rashes, respiratory issues, heartburns, and such others treated.

Apart from the fact that people are more productive when they have slept well, good sleep also prevents the advent of other health conditions like obesity, which can be a real problem for sleep-deprived individuals in the habit of sleep-eating.

Some studies have shown that 89% of adults who do not sleep enough and 55% of sleep-deprived children are likely to become obese.

Another reason poor sleep is linked to obesity is that there are some hormones, one called 'ghrelin' and another 'leptin', which directly affect sleep and appetite.

Ghrelin is known to stimulate appetite, and the body produces more of it when one has been deprived of sleep. This means that even without the problem of sleep-eating, people can still eat excessively when they have not slept enough, because of increased level of appetite and aggravated sense of hunger.

On the other hand, leptin lowers appetite and is produced to healthy levels when one has had sufficient sleep.

Experts explain that the brain of a person with no sleeping problem communicates to the body that there is sufficient energy in reserve, and therefore there is no need to feed again so soon; hence appetite is subdued.

On the overall, therefore, the best way to address the problem of insomnia or to avoid it in the first place, is by people being mindful of one's overall health.

This means eating healthy, doing reasonable exercises on a regular basis, taking care of your mental health by managing stress, and maintaining a sleep-waking routine that targets a minimum of seven hours of sleep.

Therefore, a favorable sleeping environment is bound to allow for quality sleep, a life of enhanced productivity, and general feeling of wellbeing.